H. K. Harms U. Wahn (Eds.)

Food Allergy in Infancy and Childhood

With 49 Figures and 46 Tables

Springer Verlag
Berlin Heidelberg New York
London Paris Tokyo

Professor Dr. med. H. K. Harms
Kinderklinik
Dr. v. Haunersches Kinderspital
der Universität München
Lindwurmstraße 4
8000 München 2, FRG

Professor Dr. med. U. Wahn
Kinder- und Poliklinik
Universitätsklinikum Rudolf Virchow
Standort Charlottenburg
Heubnerweg 6
1000 Berlin 19, FRG

ISBN-13: 978-3-540-50636-2 e-ISBN-13: 978-3-642-74357-3

DOI: 10. 978-3-642-74357-3

Library of Congress Cataloging-in-Publication Data.
Food allergy in infancy and childhood / H. K. Harms, U. Wahn (eds.). Bibliography, Includes index. ISBN-13: 978-3-540-50636-2 (U.S.)
1. Food allergy in infants. 2. Food allergy in children. I. Harms, H. K. II. Wahn, U.
RJ386.5.H37 1989 618.92'975 - dc19 89-6086 CIP

Typesetting and Printing: Zechnersche Buchdruckerei, Speyer
Bookbinding: Schäffer, Grünstadt
2125/3145-543210 Printed on acid-free paper

Preface

Since the beginning of the century when HAMBURGER, SCHLOSSMANN, and MORO first described food allergy in infants being fed with cow's milk, this topic has been the subject of very controversial discussions among pediatricians. The dispute is illustrated by markedly fluctuating incidence figures, ranging from denial of the disease to incidence rates up to one in ten infants. The explanation for the differing incidence figures lies in the lack of a single laboratory test which is simple as well as applicable and reliable for all clinical and immunological reactions. Even though the classic allergic hypersensitivity reactions mediated by specific IgE antibodies are relatively clearly defined, there still exist other more complex immune responses which are more difficult to recognize.

In the fall of 1987 internationally renowned experts from various fields met to define and discuss the fundamentals, organic manifestations, and the current status of diagnosis, treatment, and prevention of food allergy in childhood. The results have been collected in the volume in hand, in hopes that it will encourage more public involvement in the discussion of this illness, which is fortunately mostly transient.

Munich, Berlin; February 1989

H. K. HARMS
U. WAHN

Table of Contents

List of Contributors

Professor Dr. med. KJELL AAS	Volksentoppen P.O. Box 50 Voksenkollen 0326 Oslo 3, Norway
Dr. med. E. BARAU	Hôpital St. Vincent de Paul 74, Avenue Denfert Rocherau 75674 Paris Cedex, France
Priv. Doz. Dr. med. C. P. BAUER	Kinderklinik und Poliklinik der Technischen Universität München Kölner Platz 1 8000 München 40, FRG
Dr. med. R. M. BERTELE-HARMS	Kinderklinik Dr. v. Haunersches Kinderspital der Universität München Lindwurmstraße 4 8000 München 2, FRG
Dr. med. JEAN BOUSQUET	Service des Maladies Respiratoires Centre Hospitalier Regional de Montpellier Hopital l'Aiguelongue Montpellier, France
Professor Dr. med. LUISA BUSINCO	Department of Pediatrics Allergy and Clinical Immunology Division University La Sapienza Rome, Italy

Dr. med.
ARNALDO CANTANI

Department of Pediatrics
Allergy and Clinical Immunology Division
University La Sapienza
Rome, Italy

Dr. med.
C. DUPONT

Hôpital St. Vincent de Paul
74, Avenue Denfert Rochereau
75674 Paris Cedex, France

Dr. med.
JOSEPH EGGER

Kinderklinik
Dr. v. Haunersches Kinderspital
der Universität München
Lindwurmstraße 4
8000 München 2, FRG

Dr. med.
L. M. FAIRCLOUGH

Department of Immunology
Institute of Child Health
30, Guilford Street
London, WC1N 1EH, UK

Dr. med.
PAOLO G. GIAMPIETRO

Department of Pediatrics
Allergy and Clinical Immunology Division
University La Sapienza
Rome, Italy

Professor Dr. med.
H. K. HARMS

Kinderklinik
Dr. v. Haunersches Kinderspital
der Universität München
Lindwurmstraße 4
8000 München 2, FRG

Dr. med.
DAVID J. HILL

Allergy-Clinical Immunology Unit
Royal Children's Hospital
Melbourne, Australia

Dr. med.
ARNE HØST

Department of Pediatrics
Odense University Hospital
5000 Odense C, Denmark

Dr. med. IRÉNE JAKOBSSON	Department of Pediatrics Malmö General Hospital Malmö, Sweden
Professor Dr. med. MAX KJELLMANN	Department of Pediatrics Faculty of Health Sciences Linköpings University 581 85 Linköping, Sweden
Dr. med. S. LAU	Kinder- und Poliklinik Universitätsklinikum Rudolf Virchow Standort Charlottenburg Heubnerweg 6 1000 Berlin 19, FRG
Dr. med. Y. MARIA	Service de Médecine D Immuno-allergologie Hôpital de Brabois Vandoeuvre-Les-Nancy 54511, France
Dr. med. PAOLO MEGLIO	Department of Pediactrics Allergy and Clinical Immunology Division University La Sapienza Rome, Italy
Dr. med. FRANCOISE B. MICHEL	Service des Maladies Respiratoires Centre Hospitalier Regional de Montpellier Hopital l'Aiguelongue Montpellier, France
Dr. med. P. MOLKHOU	Hôpital St. Vincent de Paul 74, Avenue Denfert Rochereau 75674 Paris Cedex, France
Professor Dr. med. D. A. MONERET- VAUTRIN	Service de Médecine D Immuno-allergologie Hôpital de Brabois 54500 Vandoeuvre-Les-Nancy, France

Professor Dr. med. C. H. L. Rieger	Abt. Pneumologie und Immunologie Zentrum für Kinderheilkunde der Philipps-Universität Deutschhausstraße 12 3550 Marburg, FRG
Dr. med. L. Salmenperä	Children's Hospital 00290 Helsinki, Finland
Professor Dr. med. Hugh A. Sampson	Department of Pediatrics Division of Immunology John Hopkins University School of Medicine Baltimore, Maryland, USA
Dr. med. E. Savilahti	Children's Hospital 00290 Helsinki, Finland
Professor Dr. med. Martin Stern	Universitätskinderklinik Gastrointestinal and Nutrition Group Martinistraße 52 2000 Hamburg 20, FRG
Priv. Doz. Dr. med. Stephan Strobel	Department of Immunology Institute of Child Health 30, Guilford Street London, WC1N 1EH, UK
Dr. med. V.-M. Tainio	Children's Hospital 00290 Helsinki, Finland
Professor Dr. med. R. Urbanek	Universitäts-Kinderklinik Mathildenstraße 1 7800 Freiburg, FRG
Professor Dr. med. U. Wahn	Universitätsklinikum Rudolf Virchow Standort Charlottenburg Heubnerweg 6 1000 Berlin 19, FRG

Biochemical Characteristics of Food Allergens

K. Aas

Introduction

This discussion is concerned only with IgE-mediated allergy and natural allergens found in food. It does not take into consideration possible antigenicity of additives used for preservation, flavoring, or food-cosmetic purposes.

Definition of Terms

Scientific as well as clinical work in allergy must satisfy strict criteria as to specificity and precision. It is therefore necessary to be specific and precise with respect to the terms used. *Allergy* refers to hypersensitivity reactions caused by immune reactions that are harmful to the tissues or disruptive of the physiology of the host. The immune reaction triggers complex biochemical and/or inflammatory sequences which result in clinical symptoms. The symptoms depend on the degree of reactivity of the involved tissue receptors and of the effector cells. An *allergen* is an antigenic molecule that takes part in the immune reaction which results in allergy. A food allergen, for instance, is an allergen found in food. The *allergic source* is the substance that contains allergens. And an *immunogen* is a molecule, or part of it, that is able to initiate the proliferation of immunocompetent lymphocytes or to trigger the synthesis of specific antibodies.

Food Allergens Are (Mostly) Proteins

All natural allergens thus far known to react with IgE antibodies have been shown to be proteins. Many of these are glycoproteins, which means that they contain one or more sugar molecules in addition to the amino acids [1–6].

A protein is made up mainly of a number of amino acids bound together in peptide linkages, with or without a few additional carbohydrate residues in the primary structure. Each amino acid is characterized by its side chain – a chemically active site with a certain physiochemical power. Side chains contribute to the final shape and the power field of the molecule, as does any carbohydrate residue present. The chain or sequence of amino acids is twisted and is given its final shape through conformational changes due to the chemical forces between the side chains, which then fold the molecule into its tertiary structure. Chemical forces from outside also influence the final shape and the net chemical power of the molecule.

The amino acids can be said, as it were, to represent letters in a *chemical alphabet* containing a total of 20 different such letters. Carbohydrate molecules inserted in the amino acid chain act as additional letters. Combinations of these chemical letters in different ways create a multitude of words (peptide fragments) and phrases (proteins) in the language of protein chemistry. Some of the words are made by the amino acid "letters" as found in the original sequence of the chain; these are referred to as *sequential* denominators. Others are made when amino acid "letters" that are remote in the primary sequence chain are brought close together by folding of the chain. The latter are termed *conformational* denominators.

The complex mixture of proteins found in allergen sources and in extracts of allergenic foods can be demonstrated by a number of techniques, such as sodium dodecyl sulfate polyacrylamide gel electrophoresis (SDS-PAGE), isoelectrofocusing (IEF), PAGE or starch gel electrophoresis with immunoprinting, and crossed radioimmunoelectrophoresis (CRIE). A wide variety of modifications of these and similar methods have been used, and new methods are being invented. We can rightly speak of "immunoacrobatics" in this connection. Progress in protein separation methods has been an important propagator in this field of immunology, and immunology has propagated progress in protein separation and characterization. Many possibilities have been opened for those interested. This is not to say, however, that this is easy work. On the contrary, it is a demanding, tedious, and time-consuming process full of challenges, problems, and pitfalls.

Major, Intermediate, and Minor Allergens

Only one or very few of the several proteins found in a given allergen source act as essential allergens in the majority of patients allergic to the substance. The most important ones are called major allergens. Less important allergens are called intermediate or minor allergens, statistically as the case may be. It should be kept in mind that a so-called minor allergen may play a major role in rare individual patients. CRIE can be used to specify these categories more precisely; in such case, a CRIE reference system must be included in order to promote meaningful communication [7]. *A major allergen* is defined as one that binds IgE antibodies in at least 50% of sera from all the patients allergic to the substance, and that shows strong binding in at least 25% of the sera. *A minor allergen* binds IgE antibodies in not more than 10% of the sera from the same patient population. Allergens with binding capacities between these two are referred to as *intermediate allergens.*

Most, if not all, allergen sources seem to contain several distinct allergens of major, intermediate, or minor importance. They also contain an additional number of antigens which have not been shown to bind IgE antibodies. Egg white in hen's egg, for example, is a complex mixture of at least 20 distinct proteins, but only four or five of these are thought to be allergenic [8, 9]. It is possible and even likely that any one of the so-called non-IgE-binding antigens does bind IgE antibody in the serum of some rare individual who has not yet been studied in this respect.

Blands et al. [10] demonstrated 40 antigens in wheat flour, 18 of which were able to bind IgE, and three of which were considered to be major allergens. Theobald et al. [11], in a study of the sera from patients with "bakers asthma," concluded that IgE and IgG antibodies seemed to react with the same components in wheat. A clear-cut distinction between antigens and allergens was not obtained in their study. These studies were concerned with inhalant allergies to flour, however, and the results are not necessarily applicable to cereals in food. The majority of individuals reacting to wheat dust tolerate wheat in food because the most important allergens are destroyed through the process of making food from the flour.

Cow's milk contains more than 25 distinct proteins that may act as antigens in man, and a few more antigenic characteristics may arise during the intestinal passage. When absorbed, the antigenic molecules result in antibody production. The immunogenicity and antigenicity differ from protein to protein and seem to depend on host factors as well as on a combination of genetic, environmental, and adjuvant factors. Increased absorption results in a more prominent immune response and in higher serum concentrations of antibodies to milk components. Most of the antibodies do no harm. They are only innocent waste products - in a way, comparable to the sewage from the immunocompetent cell populations in the host.

According to several investigators, the most important allergens are found in β-lactoglobulin (60%–80% of cow's milk allergic patients), casein (60%), lactalbumin (50%), and bovine serum albumin (50%). Others claim that bovine serum albumin, casein, and bovine γ-globulin rank as the most common.

What Makes a Protein an Allergen?

During the past several years many allergen sources have been studied. A wide variety of allergens have been isolated and characterized, at least in part.

One may ask why some proteins act as strong allergens while others in the same food do not. For some allergen sources one may get the impression that the proteins found in the highest concentration are most likely to become allergens, but this is not consistently the case. Casein, for instance, is by far the most prominent protein in cow's milk but is not as important in allergy as β-lactoglobulin, which represents approximately 10% of the total protein. Ovalbumin in hen's egg constitutes more than half of the total protein in the egg white and is the most important allergen. Lysozyme, however, is a very weak allergen although it represents as much as 3.5%—10% of the total protein. Theoretically, there may be special physicochemical traits that are important for the transport of the molecule through living membranes, for passage of biochemical barriers, or for phagocyte handling without being directly related to antigenicity. Genetic host factors are probably as important as the molecular structure [4].

It has not been possible to specify any physiochemical feature that is characteristic for major allergens, apart from their being proteins with a molecular weight usually of between 10000 und 100000 daltons.

Those who study the classical scientific literatur regarding this may easily become confused or misled. As evaluated today, some of the earlier documentation has been confirmed, some has been shown to be only partially true, and some has been dismissed as incorrect. At one time (1960–1970) it was claimed, for example, that sugar moieties and

N-glycosidic bonding elements were mandatory for allergenic activity. To study this one must work with completely pure allergen systems, however *N*-glycosidic bond theory resulted from generalizations based on studies with impure systems. Many researchers have fallen into such pitfalls. Using a pure system we could show in 1971 that *N*-glycosidic bonds are by no means necessary for the allergic reaction as such. This does not exclude the role in other allergens of carbohydrate side chains in combination with those of certain amino acids. The importance of carbohydrate moieties has, for instance, recently been demonstrated for the allergenicity of honeybee venom phospholipase A_2 [12].

On the other hand, IgE molecules may also become bound to carbohydrate side chains in a nonspecific way. This is typical for so-called lectins (not to be discussed here) and is of clinical importance because it results in a number of false-positive diagnoses particularly in patients with a high total IgE concentration in the serum.

Denaturation and Digestion

Identification of allergens in a given food starts with a crude extract of the substance. This involves the risk that some allergenic components are not represented in the extract, either in their origional form or at all. Some may be insoluble and become lost in the sediment; others may be present in an altered form. Also, denaturation or inactivation of IgE binding may occur during the preparation of the extract. This occurs, for example, with some fruit allergens, as has been demonstrated by BJØRKSTEN et al. [13].

Furthermore, the process of fractionation and isolation of protein molecules involves great risks of inducing alterations in the conformation and charges of some of the molecules in question. The molecular folding and charge of proteins are influenced by forces exerted on them from the environmental and other proteins. Dilution itself may induce marked changes.

It is likely that isolation and dilution induce some changes of the allergenic molecules which one attempts to purify. When one has at last been able to isolate an allergen with all signs of immunological homogeneity, one may detect that the material is further separated in an electrical field when using a medium and buffer of the right kind (or the wrong kind, as one may see it). Such so-called *isoallergens* are antigenically identical moleculels that migrate slightly differently in an electrical field. They may well represents the same original molecules but have been changed slightly as to conformation and charge during the separation manipulations. The changes do not, however, affect the antigenic sites.

Questions about the degree of resistance to denaturation and digestion are especially important for food allergens. This is indicated by clinical observations. Many patients react fiercely, for example, to fresh but not to cooked apples, carrots, or potatoes. Bakers often get allergic asthma or allergic rhinitis as an occupational disease from inhaling flour dust, but they tolerate the same cereals in food. Many of the allergens in question may be very susceptible to denaturation during the preparation of food. Regarding allergens in apples, for instance, inactivation may occur as soon as the apple is cut and crushed. The fruit contains phenolic compounds and enzymes which are activated quickly upon manipulation. Phenols combine with proteins by oxidation and hydrogen bonding, resulting in denaturation and alterations of the antigenic properties of some molecules. Apple allergens could, however, be extracted in active form with media containing agents which inhibit the phenol-protein reactions [13].

On the other hand, however, such substances as hen's eggs, peanuts, nuts, peas, fish, and other seafood elicit allergic reactions almost irrespective of how the food is prepared. They may provoke allergic reactions even when found as steam droplets from the food being cooked or fried.

Thus, the allergenic epitopes in some food allergens are inactivated by denaturation and digestion while others are not affected and maintain their allergenic activity. This brings us to an essential point in the discussion of the biochemistry of food allergens.

Epitopes (Antigenic/Allergenic Determinants)

The antibody (or immune receptor of an immunocompetent lymphocyte) binds specifically to a very limited part of the antigenic molecule. This binding site is called an *epitope* or *antigenic determinant.* In this paper, *allergenic epitope* refers to an epitope in the IgE system. All proteins may be considered as complex mosaics of epitopes, comparable in the above analogy to short or long words in the language of protein chemistry. Some features may be decisive, others less so, as seen from the viewpoint of the antibody. Some components act only as necessary spacing elements keeping the essential denominators at an optimal distance from each other; others take part through more or less essential binding forces.

The number of allergenic epitopes that are accessible for the specific antibodies, and their binding dynamics, may be the factors which determine the potency of the particular allergen.

Cross-reactivities

A number of the proteins present in a given food may have some epitopes in common. This accounts for immunological cross-reactivities between different proteins within a given food and between different related foods. For example, patients allergic to the major allergen (allergen M) in codfish also react to haddock and carp white muscle proteins, which also contain allergen M. In fish allergy some patients react to all fish species tested, whereas others exhibit a marked species differentiation [14, 15].

Cross-reactivities are also found between eggs of different birds [11] or between different seafoods [15] and many other foods within the same order. Cross-reactivities are also found between certain pollen and vegetables or fruits [16, 17].

Conformational and Sequential Epitopes

Most epitopes are conformational. They result from the folding of the molecule which brings together important amino acids originally found at different sites in the primary amino acid sequence chain. Denaturation of the protein usually alters the folding and breaks up this kind of epitope. Laboratory manipulation during protein fractionation may have similar effects, making it difficult to identify conformational epitopes. It is still difficult to synthesize such epitopes.

A number of epitopes are sequential. They are organized from a number of amino acids (with or without sugar moieties) as found in the original linear sequence. This type of epitope often remains unchanged after denaturation of the protein and may be left untouched by enzymes not specific for amino acid bonds present within the epitope itself. Sequential epitopes thus lend themselves much more easily to identification and synthetization.

The Codfish Allergen Model

A sequential epitope representative for a major allergen would provide a wonderful substance for molecular research into the immunology of allergy. This was what I, myself, thought when I was occupied with this kind of research – as an incidental feature during my clinical service in pediatric department. I wanted a model for investigation of what makes an allergen an allergen, but nothing was known about the composition and structure of allergens.

It was a 7-month-old infant who presented me with a suitable model. This was a boy admitted to my department with severe atopic symptoms and who had been breast fed. We could demonstrate that he was excessively sensitive to fish, with quite fierce reactions whenever his mother had eaten fish, herself. The allergenic molecules in question had resisted cooking (denaturation), followed by digestion (proteolysis) in the mother's intestines, passage through several membranes (to the breast milk), and a second digestion in the infant's intestines. They were still active upon reaching reaginic antibodies in various tissues in the infant. From these observations, the allergenic molecules in question had to be associated with sequential units of amino acids and could probably be found in rather short fragments. Here, then, was the model allergen.

I selected codfish for the purpose and started a tedious protein fractionation and purification process, going through quite a number of trials and failures before succeeding. Codfish contains one major allergen (allergen M) found in the white muscle tissues. All codfish-allergic patients whom I have seen react to this allergen. Codfish white muscle also contains other intermediate and minor allergens, as does the blood serum of the fish. In the most sensitive patient systems the purified allergen was extremely potent. It provoked marked local whealing reactions in passive transfer, or PRAUSNITZ-KÜSTNER (PK) tests in concentrations corresponding to less than 10000 molecules injected into the sensitized sites. Double-blind food challenges with microgram quantities given to the PK test recipients provoked similar reactions. The latter experiments confirmed that the purified allergen was also absorbed in an active form through normal adult intestines. The major allergen is heat stable and quite resistant to proteolytic digestion and denaturation procedures. This supported the idea that the allergenic activity may be found in a linear sequence.

The purified allergen turned out to be a valuable tool for further work in basic as well as clinical investigations into the immunology of allergy. It was shown, for example, that most of the IgG antibodies to codfish in patients' sera reacted with other proteins than the major allergen in question. Furthermore, only a few of the IgG antibodies which bound to the allergenic molecule reacted with the same epitope as did IgE antibodies. Other IgG antibodies reacted with quite different parts of the same molecule. This is an important point in discussions about the role played by so-called "blocking antibodies." It appears that only those blocking antibodies that react with the allergenic epitope as such are likely to affect the in vivo synthesis of the IgE antibodies in question; they could thus be referred to as "allergenic epitope blocking antibodies."

Characterization of an Allergenic Epitope

The amino acid sequence of the purified allergen was analyzed. This provided enough material to propose the hypothetical model for a sequential allergenic determinant (IgE-binding epitope), presented during the 1975 Nobel Symposium in Stockholm [3]. The hypothetical model has since then been substantiated and confirmed. It is based on the assumption that the epitope may be formed by a few critical amino acid side chains found in a sequence, but allowing for one or several amino acids acting only as rather indifferent spacers keeping the critical amino acids at the optimal distance from each other.

Furthermore, at that time it had become evident that the biological reaction in IgE-mediated allergy was brought about when the allergen bound two IgE antibody molecules on the surface of mast cells or basophiles. To be allergenically active the allergen had to have at least two accessible allergenic determinants, probably of identical composition.

Assuming this, the molecule in question could have six (or even more) allergenic determinants (IgE-binding epitopes) composed by two closely connected carboxylic side chains (Asp + Glu) kept at a critical distance from the basic residue (Lys). According to this, the sequences (-Asp-Glu-Leu-Lys-), (-Asp-Glu-Asp-Lys-), and possibly (-Asp-Asp-x-Lys) offered themselves as particularly interesting candidates. The same constellations could probably also occur as conformational units (Fig. 1). Short enzymatic cleavage products from the native allergen M resulted in peptides containing Asp-Glu-Leu-Lys and Asp-Glu-Asp-Lys, which were allergenically active.

Further investigation of this has been carried out by my former colla-

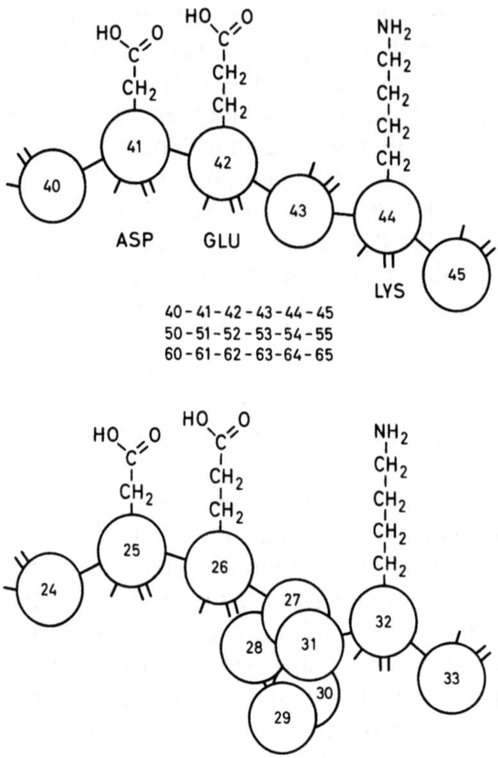

Fig. 1. Sequential and conformational combinations of amino acids thought to form essential allergenic epitopes of the major allergen (allergen M) of codfish

borator S. Elsayed, now at another laboratory in Norway. He has shown that the region composed of residues 41–64 of allergen M encompasses three of the tetrapeptides described, kept apart by two segments of six variable amino acid residues. Elsayed and coworkers produced synthetic peptides corresponding to the peptides in question. This short synthetic peptide bound IgE antibodies in the sera from codfish-allergic patients. The peptide also interfered with rabbit antiserum IgG antibodies to allergen M [18, 19]. It was the defined epitope that counted; the nature of the interspacing amino acids appeared to be without significance.

Implications for Future Research

At least two of the epitopes in question are necessary for the binding to IgE antibodies in the biological tests of allergy to codfish. To act as an immunogen for IgE antibody synthesis, however, probably only one epitope is sufficient - with or without a carrier substance. A carrier substance may be provided by the host itself, e.g., as serum albumin or heparin. In any case, extremely small fragments containing one epitope might suffice for sensitization of a disposed individual. It is therefore not likely that sensitization depends on the degree of permeability of the gut but rather on a combination of genetic and adjuvant factors in the host.

The availability of synthetic peptides that represent the allergenic determinants of natural allergens may open new fields for studies of IgE-mediated immunology. They may prove valuable in efforts to unveil mechanisms of induction as well as suppression of the immune responses in question. There is, however, no room for generalization. The codfish allergen model functions only for certain limited aspects of our many scientific problems. Other food allergens may behave in quite different ways at different levels of immune responsiveness and responses. It is surprising to me, however, that the codfish allergen model remains - after 12 years - the only one in which important epitopes have been defined. There are many other food allergens that most probably contain sequential epitopes which could also be defined. Since the allergenic activity of hen's egg white, peas, and fish is unaffected by cooking an digestion in human intestines, these foods probably contain major allergens with sequential epitopes. It is wise initially to select such material for purification and characterization purposes.

Allergens in the egg white of hen's egg are tempting material for such studies. In fact, more than 75 years have elapsed since SCHLOSS indicated this through his elegant investigations of the biochemistry of egg white allergens [20]. Availability of synthetic epitopes representing ovalbumin reacting with human IgE antibodies may provide tools for important research at the very basis of allergic immune reactions in general. I am pleased to know that such work is being carried out at present. Indeed, we need much more knowledge on this subject for all kinds of allergens, and particularly so in the confusing field of intolerance and allergy to food.

The physician is accustomed to thinking about allergy specificity with respect to allergen source. We need now to think about allergy specificity with respect to allergens on the molecular level. Furthermore, in research we must be concerned with allergen epitope specificity. To make progress in this research we need to work with pure and well-characterized preparations of allergens and epitopes.

Do not waste pure thoughts on impure preparations!

References

1. Bleumink E (1970) Food allergy. The chemical nature of the substances eliciting symptoms. World Rev Nutr Diet 12:505-570
2. King TP (1976) Chemical and biological properties of some atopic allergens. Adv Immunol 23:77-105
3. Aas K (1976) Common characteristics of major allergens. In: Johansson SGO, Strandberg K (ed) Molecular and biological aspects of the acute allergic reaction. Plenum, New York, 3-19
4. Aas K (1978) What makes an allergen an allergen. Allergy 33:3-14
5. Aas K (1980) Die Natur der Allergene. Die gelben Hefte 20:77-85
6. Brostoff J, Challacombe SJ (ed) (1987) Food allergy and intolerance. Bailliere Tindall, London
7. Aukrust L, Aas K (1977) A reference system in crossed radioimmunoelectrophoresis. Scand J Immunol 6:1093-1095
8. Hoffman DR (1983) Immunochemical identification of the allergens in egg white. J Allergy Clin Immunol 71: 481-186
9. Langeland T, Aas K (1987) Allergy to hen's egg white: clinical and immunological aspects. In: Brostoff J, Challacombe SJ (eds) Food allergy and intolerance. Bailliere Tindall, London pp 367-374
10. Blands J, Diamant B, Kallos P, Kallos-Deffner L, Løwenstein H (1976) Flour allergy in bakers. I. Identification of allergenic fractions in flour and comparison of diagnostic methods. Int Arch Allergy Appl Immunol 52:392-406
11. Theobald K, Thiel H, Kallweit C, Ulmer W, König W (1986) Detection of proteins in wheat flour extracts that bind human IgG, IgE, and mouse monoclonal antibodies. J Allergy Clin Immunol 78:470-477
12. Weber A, Schroder H, Thalberg K, Marz L (1987) Specific interaction of IgE antibodies with a carbohydrate epitope of honey bee venom phospholipase A2. Allergy 42:464-470
13. Bjørksten F, Halmepuro L, Hannuksela M, Lahti A (1980) Extraction and properties of apple allergens. Allergy 35:671-677
14. Aas K (1987) Fish allergy and the codfish allergen model. In: Brostoff J, Challacombe SJ (eds) Food allergy and intolerance. Bailliere Tindall, London pp 356-366
15. Aas K (1966) Studies of hypersensitivity to fish. Allergological and serological differentiation between various species of fish. Int Arch Allergy 30:257-267
16. Lehrer SB (1986) The complex nature of food antigens: studies of cross-reacting Crustacea allergens. Ann Allergy 57:267-272
17. Dreborg S, Foucard T (1983) Allergy to apple, carrot and potato in children with birch allergy. Allergy 38:167-172
18. Elsayed S, Apold J (1983) Immunochemical analysis of cod fish allergen M: locations of the immunoglobulin binding sites as demonstrated by the native and synthetic peptides. Allergy 38:449-459
19. Elsayed S (1983) The native and synthetic peptides of codfish allergen M. A short review. In: Bostrøm H, Epne H, Ljungstedt N (eds) Theoretical and clinical aspects of allergic diseases. Almqvist and Wiksell, Stockholm pp 237-253
20. Schloss OM, Worthen TW (1969) The permeability of the gastro-enterologic tract of infants to undigested protein. Am J Dis Child ii:342-360

Mucosal Passage and Handling of Food-Protein Antigens*

M. Stern

The occurrence of cow's milk allergy (CMA) was reported early in this century [29] as an example of food-protein allergy during early infancy in man. Using indirect immunological methods, different researchers demonstrated that food proteins in young infants were taken up either undigested [35] or incompletely digested [13]. For a long time after this early work, increased uptake of incompletely digested food protein material was thought to constitute the major pathogenetic factor in the development of food allergy. The results of animal studies and a few human studies have provided new insights into the complicated interrelation between mucosal barrier elements and the gut-associated lymphoid tissue (GALT) and into processes such as the mucosal handling and transmucosal passage of food proteins. Clinical methods have made possible the definition of the relative allergenic potential of single cow's milk proteins (Table 1; for references see [29]).

Uptake of Intact Food Proteins is a Physiological Phenomenon

The concept of gastrointestinal immunophysiology is founded on morphological studies demonstrating that macromolecules can penetrate the gastrointestinal mucosa by various routes. These include: (a) microfold cells ("M cells") overlying Peyer's patches, (b) intact enterocytes (endocytosis/exocytosis), and (c) intercellular gaps ("tight" junctions). These routes make possible different steps of interaction between the ingested protein and gastrointestinal elements. These forms of interaction and intraluminal degradation are referred to as "gastrointestinal handling" of food protein antigens. The intact macromolecule can be traced from the gut surface to the subepithelial level of lymphoid folli-

* Supported by Deutsche Forschungsgemeinschaft DFG Ste 305

Table 1. Cow's milk proteins functioning as allergens

Protein	Concentration in cow's milk (g/dl)	Allergenicity in man
Casein	2.5	++
β-Lactoglobulin	0.3	+++
α-Lactalabumin	0.07	+
Bovine γ-globulin	0.06	+
Bovine serum albumin	0.03	+

cles [16]. This does not imply any pathological condition, but it may contribute to the pathophysiology of food allergy or bacterial diarrhoea if the physiological balance between antigen exposure, handling and presentation to GALT is disturbed.

Food Protein Handling by the Gut Modifies Allergenicity

The handling of food proteins has been investigated using various animal models both with and without immunization of the animals by the respective antigen. Different effects are possible on the relative allergenicity of food proteins. First, the protein may escape handling and proteolysis, and allergenically intact food protein may be detected in the gastrointestinal contents of the small bowel [12]. Appreciable amounts of the cow's milk protein β-lactoglobulin (BLG) may be detected even in the blood of neonatal guinea pigs, an uptake process that ceases after the 6th postnatal day [33]. Postnatal maturation was clearly shown to determine this uptake of intact food protein. Second, handling may lead to protein breakdown products that retain part of the original allergenicity [6, 36]; in some cases, proteolysis may even generate new antigens from bovine milk proteins [26]. Third, proteolytic fragments of proteins such as bovine serum albumin (BSA) may exhibit tolerogenic properties instead of allergenic ones [4, 14]. And fourth, the food protein may be broken down rapidly to small peptides and amino acids, so that no transmucosal passage of immunologically active food protein fragments can take place. In studies using soy proteins in preruminant calves [11, 24], experimentally induced anaphylaxis was shown to diminish the hydrolysis of intestinal food protein. In anmimals hypersensitive to soy, more dietary antigen survived proteolysis and was able to perpetuate the adverse reaction.

In a series of experiments using the gut sacs of adult nonimmune rats as an in vitro model [27], various aspects of mucosal food protein handling were investigated, including binding to the mucus coat, breakdown, and uptake into the serosal gut sac compartment (Fig. 1). Binding and uptake of BSA and BLG were closely correlated. Both processes were nonspecific and nonsaturable, unlike other physiological transport phenomena. A consistent finding was that much more BLG was bound and taken up than BSA. Thus, different proteins were clearly shown to undergo differential handling by the gut. This may help to explain differences in relative allergenicity. Gel filtration experiments were carried out to study the breakdown of food proteins in detail (Fig. 2). By this technique it was shown that BLG is broken down much more readily in to small peptide fragments, compared to BSA

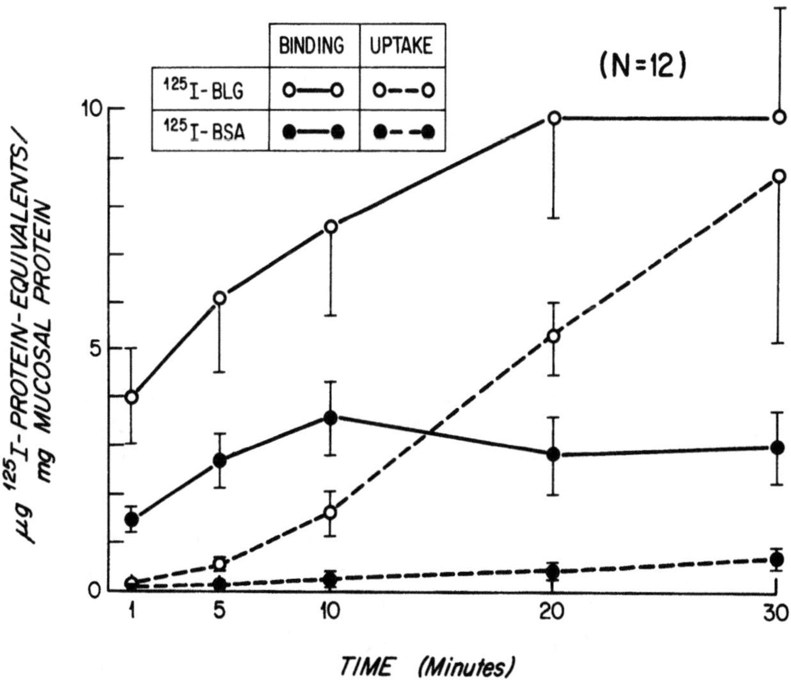

Fig. 1. Binding and uptake of ^{125}I-labelled BSA and BLG by adult rat gut sacs from jejunum. Binding and uptake are correlated. Binding and uptake of ^{125}I-labelled BLG exceed binding and uptake of ^{125}I-labelled BSA. (From [27])

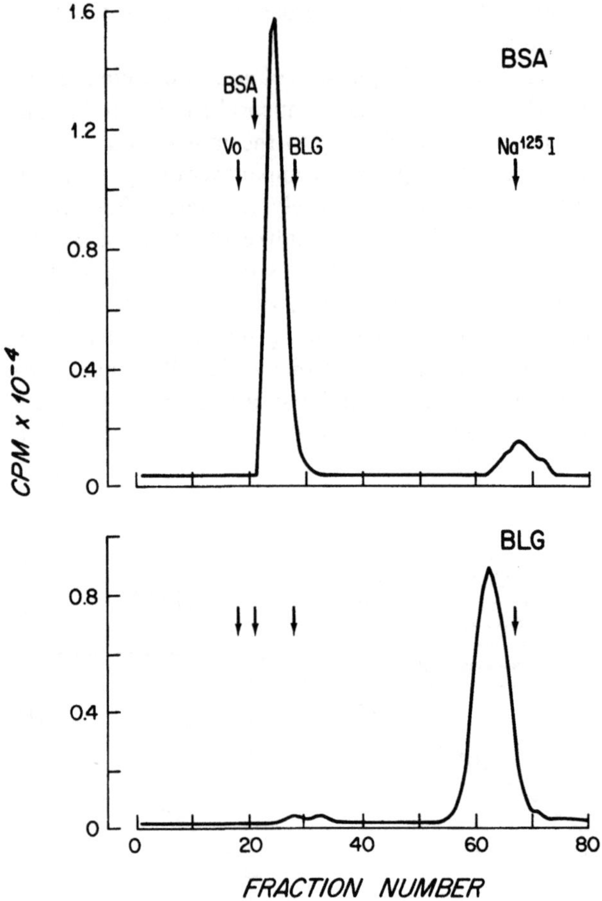

Fig. 2. Gel filtration profiles of mucosal scrapings after 10 min incubation with ^{125}I-labelled BSA and BLG. Calibration is indicated by *arrows*. ^{125}I-labelled BLG is much more rapidly broken down to small fragments; mol. wt. <4000. (From [27])

which retains most of this original molecular size during incubation. It was also shown that the size and structure fragments after intestinal handling of different cow's milk proteins influence mucus coat binding and uptake of the respective food antigens. The way in which different steps of food protein handling are ionvolved in food hypersensitivity is an issue that must be dealt with by future experiments. Gastrointestinal handling of food antigens appears to be closely interrelated with local immune reactions of GALT to these antigens.

Nonspecific Gastrointestinal Mucosal Barrier Protects Against Transmucosal Passage of Intraluminal Macromolecular Antigens

The gastrointestinal tract is not only an organ system for nutrient digestion and absorption but also a site of confrontation. During early infancy, the gastrointestinal tract must face many foreign, potentially allergenic substances that have been ingested (e.g. microorganisms, food proteins). After surviving digestion and handling in a more or less modified form, these substances come into contact with phagocytes and immunocompetent cells of the specific immunological host defence system, represented by GALT, which comprises 25% of gut mucosal tissue. Taken together, luminal and mucosal nonspecific mechanisms of antigen encounter and modification prior to presentation to GALT support the concept of a nonspecific gastrointestinal barrier against the uncontrolled and overwhelming transmucosal penetration of foreign macromolecules ([32]; Table 2). Various organs of the gastrointestinal tract are involved, but of paramount importance is the composition of the small-intestinal surface, which consists of the mucus coat [5, 23] and the microvillus membrane (MVM) of villus enterocytes.

Even after antigen encounter with GALT, there are mechanisms of antigen elimination and exclusion that combine nonspecific factors such as phagocytosis and specific immunological factors such as immune complex formation [32]. Kupffer cell mediated hepatic elimination of antigens is an example of this part of the mucosal barrier. GALT

Table 2. Elements of the nonspecific gastrointestinal mucosal barrier

Intraluminal
Proteolysis (gastric, pancreatic)
Peristalsis
Mucosal surface
Mucus coat, glycocalyx
Enterocyte
Microvillus membrane (MVM)
Lysosomal degradation
Subepithelial
Phagocytosis by macrophages
Hepatic elimination (Kupffer cells)

(From [32])

combines humoral (secretory IgA) and cell-mediated lines of immune defence against foreign macromolecules and antigens [21, 25].

Gastrointestinal Mucosal Barrier is Subject to Postnatal Maturation

Nonspecific and specific immune components of the gastrointestinal mucosal barrier are not completely developed at birth but evolve postnatally, at first encounter with food antigenic material [8]. In the experimental animal, for instance, in neonatal pigs [34], the phenomenon of gut closure to the uptake of macromolecules occurs during this period. In man, this process is more complex. Apart from the overall effect of gut closure, individual barrier elements are subject to postnatal maturation. This is true for the chemical composition and physical properties of small-intestinal mucus [23]. Immature viscosity and hydration status of the mucus coat gel layer covering the small-intestinal cellular surface may contribute to defects of local nonspecific host defence [5].

The enterocyte surface membrane (MVM) reveals distinct biochemical and biophysical changes during the newborn period in a number of animal species [17]. Lectin binding patterns, glycoprotein composition, and membrane organization and fluidity exhibit considerable immaturity during early postnatal life. In a recent series of experiments, we studied the effects of MVM immaturity on the handling, binding and uptake of food proteins in neonatal rats [28, 30]. Surface binding of cow's milk proteins to MVM from neonatal and adult rats showed increased binding of all the proteins in the neonatal preparations (Fig. 3). Binding was nonspecific, noninhibitable, and weak compared, for instance, to that of lectins. Molecular weight was clearly one, but not the only, factor determining differences in the cow's milk proteins tested. A longitudinal study revealed that the change in binding occurs early, before weaning (Fig. 4).

Antigen breakdown was not involved in the MVM model since the material bound was shown to remain intact. In the gut sac model using preparations from 18-day-old preweanling rats [28], it could be demonstrated that immature animals were not able to break down the proteins tested as completely as were adult controls. In these gut sacs from preweanling rats, there was not only decreased breakdown but also decreased binding to the complex mucus coat and, consequently, decreased of iodinated material from labelled food protein solutions into the serosal gut sac compartment [28]. It was concluded that gut sac

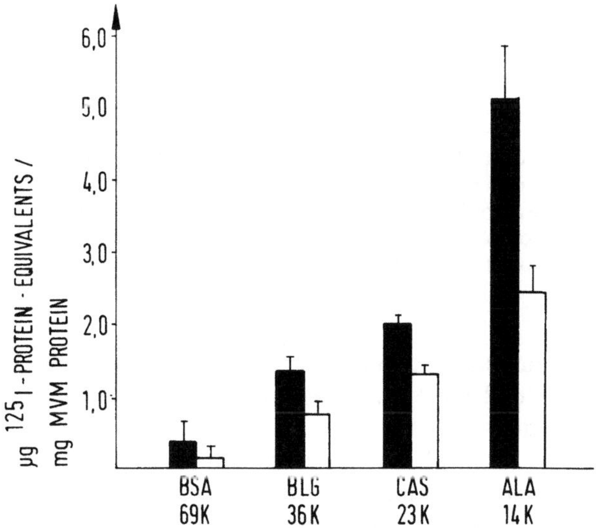

Fig. 3. Binding of ^{125}I-labelled cow's milk proteins by newborn (*shaded columns*) and adult (*unshaded columns*) rat MVM. *CAS*, Casein; *ALA*, α-lactalbumin. Newborn membranes are consistently binding more cow's milk proteins. Molecular weight (in kilodaltons) is shown at the bottom. (From [30])

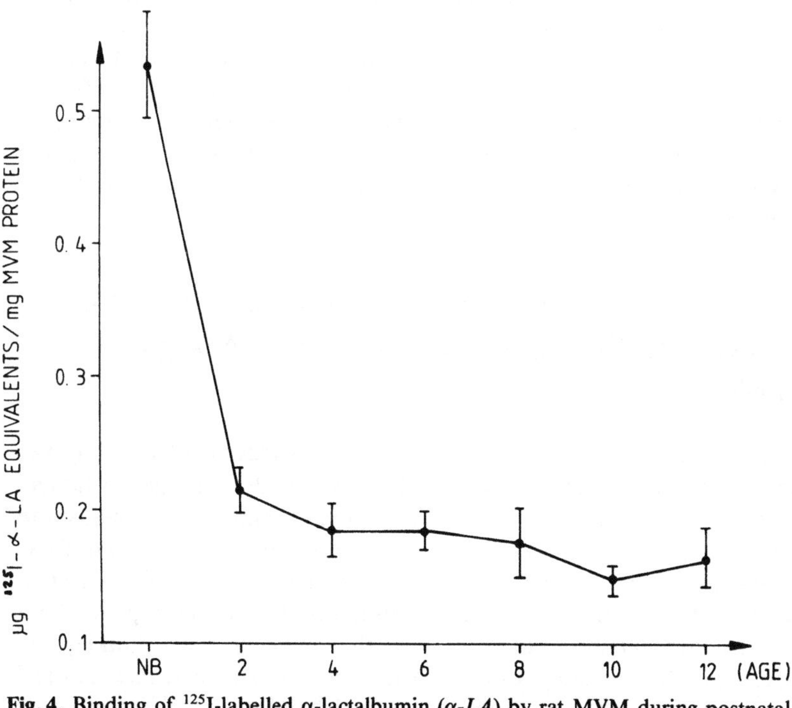

Fig. 4. Binding of ^{125}I-labelled α-lactalbumin (*α-LA*) by rat MVM during postnatal maturation (in weeks). Binding declines to adult values early, before weaning

Table 3. Effects of immaturity of gastrointestinal mucosal barrier in various animal models (whole animals, gut sacs, microvillus membranes)

Binding of food proteins to mucus coat	Decrease
Binding of food proteins to MVM	Increase
Breakdown of food proteins	Decrease
Uptake of intact food proteins	Increase
Uptake of protein fragments	Decrease

preparations contain protective elements against binding and uptake of intact food proteins. MVM from newborn animals is deficient in this protection.

As a result of the various individual events described above, intact food protein is taken up in higher quantities by immature animals, as has been shown in our laboratory [31] earlier. The effects of immaturity of the gastrointestinal mucosal barrier in different animal models are summarized in Table 3. As a consequence of these changes, neonatal animals are more exposed to intact antigenic food protein material. At this point, it can not be concluded whether this actually means any harmful effect, but it does bear harmful potential, as shown in numerous models of hypersensitivity [11, 21, 24, 33]. Gastrointestinal food allergy and increased neonatal susceptibility to gastrointestinal infection may well be connected to immaturity of the host defence system [32]. Human studies are needed to determine whether hypotheses stemming from animal work also hold true for the clinical situation in early human infancy.

Is Immaturity of the Gastrointestinal Mucosal Barrier Relevant to the Development of Food Allergy in Man?

Recent work has demonstrated that increased macromolecular uptake occurs not only in the experimental animal model but also in human preterm neonates [1, 10, 15, 20]. The degree of immaturity necessary to ascertain increased uptake varied in these reports, ranging from 29–34 weeks gestational age [10] to 36 weeks of gestation [15, 20]. Different cow's milk proteins were affected differently [15], so that a general gut closure phenomenon to the uptake of all proteins appears unlikely. Interestingly, this finding coincides with data from animal research [27] demonstrating differential gastrointestinal handling of different cow's milk proteins. Thus, some protein-specific handling and uptake mechanism must be postulated.

None of these studies reported adverse effects of increased uptake of cow's milk. There are, however, studies which show macromolecular uptake to be increased in such human pathological conditions as worm infection [19], malabsorption and food allergy [3] and malnutrition [9]. Serum food protein levels were affected by serum antibodies to the same proteins [3]. The direct pathophysiological potential of these findings remains to be investigated. Any view of the problem of food protein uptake that does ot account for simultaneous and systemic immune reactions would be incomplete and misleading. More work on nonspecific and specific factors in the transmucosal passage of food proteins is definitely needed.

Morphological work has traced food proteins and local sites of food antibody production in children with diarrhoea and cow's milk protein intolerance [2, 18]. Even in these studies it remains unclear whether these phenomena are primary or secondary. Likewise, in immediate hypersensitivity to cow's milk in children, it has been shown that cow's milk protein fragments retain their allergenic potential as regards IgE antibody production [7, 22]. It is unclear, however, whether really new allergenic epitopes are revealed or formed by proteolysis and handling of food proteins in man. Thus, the question remains as to whether immaturity of the gastrointestinal mucosal barrier is basically relevant to the development of food allergy in man. From animal models, and from some direct evidence in man, interesting concepts have evolved that suggest links between immaturity and other disturbances of the mucosal host defence, on the one hand, and the development of adverse reactions to food proteins and gastrointestinally presented antigens, on the other. The data to support these concepts must still be substantiated considerably.

References

1. Beach RC, Menzies IS, Clayden GS, Scopes JW (1982) Gastrointestinal permeability changes in the preterm neonate. Arch Dis Child 57:141–145
2. Bock SA, Remigio LK, Gordon B (1983) Immunochemical localization of proteins in the intestinal mucosa of children with diarrhea. J Allergy Clin Immunol 72:262–268
3. Dannaeus A, Inganäs M, Johansson SGO, Foucard T (1979) Intestinal uptake of ovalbumin in malabsorption and food allergy in relation to serum IgG antibody and orally administered sodium cromoglycate. Clin Allergy 9:263–270

4. Ferguson TA, Peters T, Reed R, Pesce AJ, Michael JG (1983) Immunoregulatory properties of antigenic fragments from bovine serum albumin. Cell Immunol 78:1–12
5. Forstner GG, Forstner JE (1981) Mucosal barrier and its defense mechanisms during the perinatal period. In: Lebenthal E (ed) Textbook of gastroenterology and nutrition in infancy. Raven, New York, pp 201–210
6. Gardner MLG, Lindblad BS, Burston D, Matthews DM (1983) Trans-mucosal passage of intact peptides in the guinea-pig small intestine in vivo: a reappraisal. Clin Soc 64:433–439
7. Haddad ZH, Kalra V, Verma S (1979) IgE antibodies to peptic and peptic-tryptic digests of beta-lactoglobulin: significance in food hypersensitivity. Ann Allergy 42:395–396
8. Henning SJ (1981) Postnatal development: coordination of feeding, digestion, and metabolism. Am J Physiol 241:G199–214
9. Heyman M, Boudraa G, Sarrut S, Giraud M, Evans L, Touhami M, Desjeux JF (1984) Macromolecular transport in jejunal mucosa of children with severe malnutrition: a quantitative study. J Pediatr Gastroenterol Nutr 3:357–363
10. Jakobsson I, Lindberg T, Lothe L, Axelsson I, Benediktsson B (1986) Human alpha-lactalbumin as a marker of macromolecular absorption. Gut 27:1029–1034
11. Kilshaw PJ, Slade H (1980) Passage of ingested protein into the blood during gastrointestinal hypersensitivity reactions: experiments in te preruminant calf. Clin Exp Immunol 41:575–582
12. Koritz TN, Suzuki S, Coombs RRA (1987) Antigenic stimulation with proteins of cow's milk via the oral route in guinea pigs and rats. I. Measurement of antigenically intact beta-lactoglobulin and casein in the gastrointestinal contents of duodenum, jejunum and ileum. Int Arch Allergy Appl Immunol 82:72–75
13. Lippard VW, Schloss OM, Johnson PA (1936) Immune reactions induced in infants by intestinal absorption of incompletely digested cow's milk protein. Am J Dis Child 51:562–574
14. Muckerheide A, Pesce AJ, Michael JG (1977) Immunosuppressive properties of a peptic fragment of BSA. J Immunol 119:1340–1345
15. Müller G, Bernsau I, Müller W, Weissbarth-Riedel E, Natzschka J, Rieger CHL (1986) Cow milk protein antigens and antibodies in serum of premature infants during the first 10 days of life. J Pediatr 109:869–873
16. Owen RL (1977) Sequential uptake of horseradish peroxidase by lympohoid follicle epoithelium of Peyer's patches in the normal unobstructed mouse intestine: an ultrastructural study. Gastroenterology 72:440–451
17. Pang KY, Bresson JL, Walker WA (1983) Development of the gastrointestinal mucosal barrier. Evidence for structural differences in microvillus membranes from newborn and adult rabbits. Biochim Biophys Acta 727:201–208
18. Pearson JR, Kingston D, Shiner M (1983) Antibody production to milk proteins in the jejunal mucosa of children with cow's milk protein intolerance. Pediatr Res 17:406–412
19. Reinhardt MC, Paganelli R, Levinsky R (1983) Intestinal antigen handling at mucosal surfaces in health and disease: human and experimental studies. Ann Allergy 51:311–314
20. Roberton DM, Paganelli R, Dinwiddie R et al. (1982) Milk antigen absorption in the preterm and term neonate. Arch Dis Child 57:372

21. Roberts SA, Reinhardt MC, Paganelli R et al. (1981) Specific antigen exclusion and nonspecific facilitation of antigen entry across the gut in rats allergic to food proteins. Clin Exp Immunol 45:131-136
22. Schwartz HR, Neruskar LS, Spies JR et al. (1980) Milk hypersensitivity: RAST studies using new antigens generated by pepsin hydrolysis of beta-lactoglobulin. Ann Allergy 45:242-245
23. Shub MD, Pang KY, Swann DA, Walker WA (1983) Age-related changes in chemical composition and physical properties of mucus glycoporoteins from rat small intestine. Biochem J 215:405-411
24. Sissons JW, Thurston SM (1984) Survival of dietary antigens in the digestive tract of calves intolerant to soyabean products. Res Vet Sci 37:242-246
25. Skogh T, Edebo L, Stendahl O (1983) Gastrointestinal uptake and blood clearance of antigen in the presence of IgA antibodies. Immunology 50:175-180
26. Spies JR, Stevan MA, Stein WJ et al. (1970) The chemistry of allergens. XX. New antigens generated by pepsin hydrolysis of bovine milk proteins. J Allergy 45:208-219
27. Stern M, Walker WA (1984) Food proteins and gut mucosal barrier. I. Binding and uptake of cow's milk proteins by adult rat jejenum in vitro. Am J Physiol 246:G556- 562
28. Stern M, Pang KY, Walker WA (1984) Food proteins and gut mucosal barrier. II. Differential interaction of cow's milk proteins with the mucous coat and the surface membrane of adult and immature rat jejunum. Pediatr Res 18:1252-1256
29. Stern M, Walker WA (1985) Food allergy and intolerance. Pediatr Clin North Am 32:471-492
30. Stern M, Gellermann B (1989) Food proteins and maturation of small intestinal microvillus membranes (MVM). I. Binding characteristics of cow's milk proteins and concanavalin A to MVM from newborn and adult rats. J Pediatr Gastroenterol Nutr 7:115-121
31. Udall JN, Pang K, Fritze L et al. (1981) Development of gastrointestinal musosal barrier. I. The effect of age on intestinal permeability to macromolecules. Pediatr Res 15:241-244
32. Walker WA (1987) Transmucosal passage of antigens. In: Reinhardt E, Schmidt E (eds) Food allergy. Raven, New York, pp 15-34
33. Weaver LT, Koritz TN, Coombs RRA (1987) Tolerance to orally induced anaphylactic sensitisation to cow's milk proteins and patency of the intestinal mucosa in the neonatal guinea pig. Int Arch Allergy Appl Immunol 83:220-222
34. Weström B, Svendsen J, Tagesson C (1984) Intestinal permeability to polyethyleneglycol 600 in relation to macromolecular closure in the neonatal pig. Gut 25:520-525
35. Wilson SJ, Walzer M (1935) Absorption of undigested proteins in human beings. IV. Absorption of unaltered egg protein in infants and in children. Am J Dis Child 50:49-54
36. Wright RN, Rothberg R (1971) The reactions of pepsin and pepsin-trypsin digestion products of bovine serum albumin with antisera from rabbits ingesting this protein. J Immunol 107:1410-1418

Immune Responses of the Young to Foods: Developmental Aspects of Food Allergy

S. Strobel

Introduction

The risk of developing a food-sensitive (allergic) disease is generally higher in children than it is in adults. This clinical observation highlights the importance of – as yet ill-defined – perinatal factors in the development of food-allergic diseases.

In this short review, I will outline the importance of peri- and postnatal host responses of the infant to food antigens which reach the gut-associated lymphoid tissues (GALT) directly or via the breast milk. After a brief summary of the development of neonatal immunity, I will

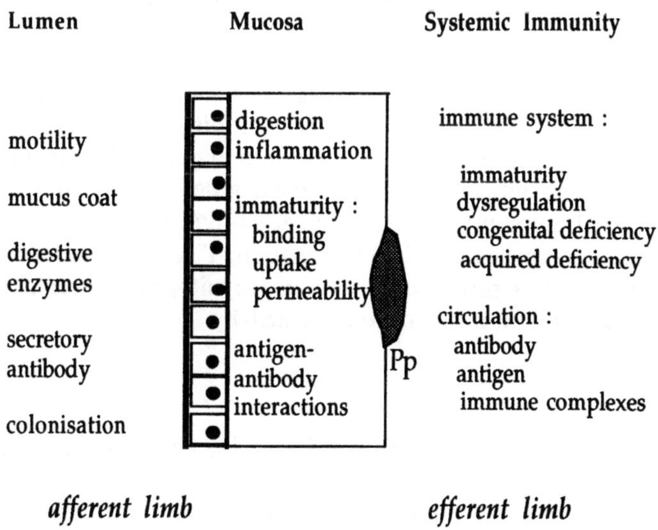

Fig. 1. Summary of factors influencing the local and systemic immune responses after oral antigen administration

deal separately with the *afferent* and the *efferent* parts of the immune response. The afferent limb involves antigen-handling and absorption mechanisms on the lumenal side of the mucosa whereas the *efferent* limb entails the immune responses initiated *after* the antigen has reached the circulation or the organised lymphoid tissues of the gut, the Peyer's patches (Fig. 1). Clinical or experimental conditions will be mentioned which are likely to modulate the induction of oral tolerance (oral tolerance defined as a specific immunological hyporesponsiveness after antigen presentation via the gut).

Immunity of the Young Infant

Humoral Immunity. B cells have been shown to be functionally immature at birth. This does affect the IgM response, which is fully mature at birth whereas IgG and IgA serum antibody responses are not. Humoral immunity reaches nearly adult levels (IgA production may still be immature) at around 2 years of age. IgG subclass responses mature at a different rate. IgG1 and IgG3 responses are present within 1st year of life whereas IgG2 and IgG4 may not have reached mature levels of responsiveness even after 2 years.

Cell-Mediated Immune Responses. In comparison to humoral immune responses, T-cell immunity is mature at birth. T-lymphocytes of fetuses of 15–16 weeks of gestation respond to major histocompatibility (HLA) and foreign antigens [1]. A clinical example to demonstrate the maturity of T-cell immunity at birth is the adult-like response to postnatal BCG (Calmette-Guérin bacillus) vaccination. T cells of the human newborn show a mature proliferative response to mitogens, a normal lymphokine production and normal cytotoxic activity.

Nonspecific Immunity of the Human Neonate

The non-specific or innate immunity of the neonate is immature at birth and affects phagocytosis, antigen presentation and the classical pathway of complement activation [2–4]. Cord blood also contains a unique suppressor cell activity [5], and these cells are able to suppress adult T-cell functions but not allogeneic (neonatal) cells [6].

Intestinal Permeability and Absorption

The gastrointestinal permeability of the premature and term newborn to intact macromolecules [7] and to inert sugar molecules [8] (e.g. lactulose, cellobiose and rhamnose) has been investigated extensively. There is still controversy as to how long the increased uptake of cow's milk antigens bovine serum albumin (BSA) and β-lactoglobulin (BLG) persists. To summarise the published evidence, it seems that the gastrointestinal permeability of the premature infant (less than 36 weeks of gestation) is uniformly increased both to high and low molecular weight marker molecules (Fig. 2).

Changes in permeability to sugars do not necessarily reflect increased macromolecular absorption, and recent evidence for an increased sugar permeability combined with a normal protein permeability during an anaphylactic response in the rat has been published [9]. Macromolecular absorption is dependent on the molecular size, structure and charge of the protein. According to a recent study [10] the overall permeability to cow's milk proteins (BLG and α-casein) may not only depend on the gestational age but could also be influenced by choice of the cow's milk protein. This work, if confirmed, would indicate an age-related, different – and mutually exclusive – pattern of mucosal permeability for two major nutritional proteins. Specific immune complex formation and maternal antibodies may have affected the results. Ethical considerations restrict studies of antigen absorption in the neonate basically to nutritional proteins (mainly cow and soya proteins). The advantage of

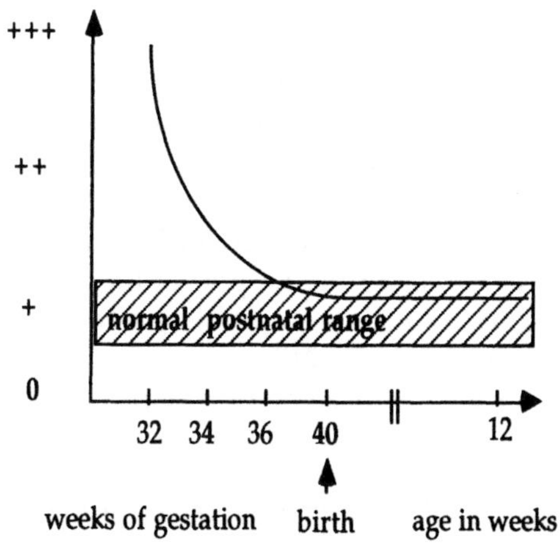

Fig. 2. Decline of mucosal permeability to proteins (BLG, BSA, etc.), mono- and disaccharides (e.g. lactulose, rhamnose, etc.) in relation to gestational age

using a normal dietary antigen is reduced by the influences of immunity transferred during birth and/or lactation.

A different approach was taken by a Swedish group [11] which measured the serum concentration of human lactalbumin. This is a protein of human milk and is taken up unaffected by local or systemic immune responses. These studies demonstrate increased levels of human lactalbumin in prematures (26–31 weeks of gestation) and are in agreement with results obtained with cow's milk proteins. Increased mucosal permeability is, however, most likely *not* sufficient to induce sensitisation without an underlying immunoregulatory abnormality. Genetic factors, for example, affecting the antigen-processing capacity and/or the immune responsiveness of the host (Ir genes), may play a more important role in the process of sensitisation.

Human Milk and the Immunity of Lactation

Breast milk is regarded as the optimal source of nutrition, and it also transfers active and passive protective immunity to the neonate. In 1892 Ehrlich [12] demonstrated that immunity can be transferred by breast milk (in mice). Later studies demonstrated that human colostrum (and milk) provides important immunity during early neonatal development [13, 14]. High levels of IgA antibodies in human milk prevent bacterial attachment which may also protect against potentially harmful immune responses to ingested antigens [15]. Human milk is also a source of common food antigens [16] which may also trigger food-allergic symptoms in the infant, and rare incidences of sensitisation via breast milk have been described [17]. I believe it still premature, however, to suggest that dietary manipulations of the mother may be helpful in preventing food-allergic disease in the neonate [18].

Breast feeding does not seem to be an important source of sensitisation in a population at risk, and it is more likely to protect the population of infants against infections and food-allergic diseases [19, 20]. There is no doubt that breast feeding reduces the number of infectious episodes during the 1st year of life, but studies questioning the protective effects against atopic diseases have been published in similar numbers (reviewed in [21]).

A study by Savilahti et al. [22] casts some doubts on the beneficial effects of prolonged breast feeding (over 3 months) on the reduction of allergic symptoms in infants at risk. It points to heredity as being the single major determining factor in the development of atopic disease.

This study also demonstrates that breast feeding reduces the diarrhoeal episodes in early infancy. Further studies are needed, and these observations *cannot* be taken as an argument against prolonged breast feeding.

Passive Transfer of Antibody and its Effects on Humoral Immunity

Placental transfer of specific antibodies protects the neonate against pathogens (experienced by the mother prior to birth) before it is capable of mounting an active humoral immune response. High levels of IgG antibodies to food antigens (mainly milk and egg) in cord sera also reflect maternal immunity. High levels of maternal anti-food antibodies correlate *slightly* with a protection against atopic (IgE-mediated) disease during the first 2 years of life [23]. In animals, circulating maternal antibodies can limit the transfer of a dietary protein from mother to newborn [24]. It remains to be established whether the reduction of "maternally processed" antigen in an experimental system has beneficial effects on the offspring in reducing the chances of subsequent sensitisation. Passively transferred maternal anti-bovine serum albumin (BSA) antibodies do not interfere with the production of anti-BSA antibodies in the human neonate [25, 26]. These findings suggest that the antibody formation against ingested antigens (IgG, IgM) occurs unaffected by the presence of circulating maternal antibodies [27]. These observations are at first glance at variance with the fact that circulating antibodies can modulate systemic immune responses to *parenterally* administered antigens (see, for example, the effects of circulating specific antibodies on the reduced 'take rate' of measles vaccinations). This highlights the important differences in immune responses after *enteral* or *systemic* antigen administration.

Specific Antibody Production of the Neonate

Ethical considerations restrict the investigations of the neonate's capacity to produce specific antibody to food antigens such as BSA or BLG. Premature infants from the 36th week of gestation are capable of producing antibodies directed against these antigens, and by 4 years of age (almost) all children have circulating antibodies against milk proteins [27, 28].

Perinatal Modulation of IgE Responses by Transfer of Antibody

Studies in humans have demonstrated that circulating maternal anti-BSA antibodies (IgG or IgM) had no effect on the child's further maturation of humoral immunity to ingested BSA [25, 27]. This may not be true for the regulation of IgE synthesis. Evidence to support a modulatory effect of IgG antibody on IgE synthesis has been presented by the late E. JARRETT and her group. In a series of experiments, stimulation of adult rats with antigens, whether injected or fed, led more often to *reduced* than enhanced IgE responses after subsequent challenge. The capacity to suppress IgE synthesis is activated by minute amounts of antigen which are frequently absorbed intact via the gastrointestinal mucosa. It was hypothesised that this would maintain the down-regulation of the IgE response in the neonatal rat [29]. Further experiments demonstrated that there is a marked suppression of IgE responsiveness in the offspring of parenterally immunised female rats, and that this state of suppression in the neonatal rat persists even when the circulating maternal antibody is no longer detectable [30]. To summarise, it seems that both specific maternal IgG and specific antigen have a profound effect on the regulation of the IgE response [31]. The existence of a similar regulating pathway for *human* IgE responses has not been established.

Regulation of the Immune Response After Antigen Ingestion (Oral Tolerance)

An antigen can be defined as a substance which elicits a specific immune response when introduced into the tissues of an individual (or an animal). Protein molecules may have several antigenic determinants, and any antigen may evoke several, not mutually exclusive, immune responses. When the antigen is administered via the gut, both systemic and mucosal immune reactions occur, resulting in induction or suppression of a particular immune response (antibody or T-cell mediated) [32, 33]. Active *immunity*, in which antigen reactive cells and specific antibody develop, must be distinguished from immunological *tolerance*, which is defined as a specific systemic hyporesponsiveness if the antigen is subsequently given parenterally [32, 34]. The phenomenon of immunological tolerance to ingested proteins (*oral tolerance*) has been studied mainly in animal models [32, 34, 35]; circumstantial evidence implies, however, that it exists in man too [36, 37].

The primary route of antigen presentation is crucial, and the subsequent immune responses may be modified, but they are rarely completely reversed as a result of further antigen exposure. Chronic, high-dose antigen exposure after initial immunisation can, however, modulate the immune responses, which has been shown in adult [38] and neonatal animals [39]. This treatment does not usually re-induce a complete state of tolerance. Preliminary evidence suggests that mice [40] immunised with ovalbumin in complete Freund's adjuvant and re-fed 1 week after immunisation show a substantial reduction of their cell-mediated immune response to ovalbumin ($p<0.01$) as well as a reduction of their serum antibody levels, although to a lesser extent ($0.05<p<0.1$; H.-J. Peng, M.W. Turner, S. Strobel, unpublished observation). These observations underline the fact that the two limbs of the immune system are under different control and are affected differently by oral antigen exposure [40].

In summary, immune responses which develop after mucosal antigen exposure are associated with stimulation of several types of immune regulatory T-lymphocytes in the GALT [41, 42]. Within the Peyer's patches and other organised lymphoid tissues of the gut, specific T helper and T suppressor cells are activated. There appears to be a dual activation of the T-lymphocytes which regulate the B-lymphocyte population; there also seems to be an induction of T helper cells for the IgA system and of suppressor cells for IgM and IgG synthesis [44]. The time of first antigen exposure is crucial and several groups have shown that the early postnatal administration of antigens can cause gastrointestinal diseases, which are probably due to cell-mediated immune responses within the gastrointestinal tract. This phenomenon has been shown in the pre-ruminant calf, in piglets and in mice [44–46].

Antigen Administration During the Neonatal Period

Clinical experience suggests a vulnerable period for potential sensitisations to foods within the first 4–8 weeks of life during the maturation of the GALT and systemic immunity of the neonate. Potentially hazardous effects of early antigen administration on the development of food-allergic disease have been investigated by studying the effects of age at first feed on the development of subsequent specific systemic immunity (in mice). Suppression (tolerance) or priming (enhancement of the immune response) of the immune system was investigated in animals which had been fed hen's albumin (OVA) at various times after birth (1–42 days). Full details of the methods and results have been published [39, 46, 47]. The findings, summarised in Fig. 3, show that animals fed at 14 and 42 days were tolerant (as expected), but that animals fed OVA between 1 and 7 days of age did *not* develop oral tolerance, and that indeed mice fed on the day of birth repeatedly and consistently developed signs of priming, both for antibodies and for cell-mediated immunity.

Antigen Exposure Before Birth

It is still not clear whether circulating maternal antigen reaches the fetal circulation or the amniotic fluid, and whether it is capable of inducing an immune response in utero. Individual reports of sensitisation prior to birth do not address this question, and anti-idiotypic priming cannot be ruled out or confirmed at this stage [49].

In order to control antigen administration and delivery we exposed individual fetuses to OVA by intra-amniotic injection during a laparo-

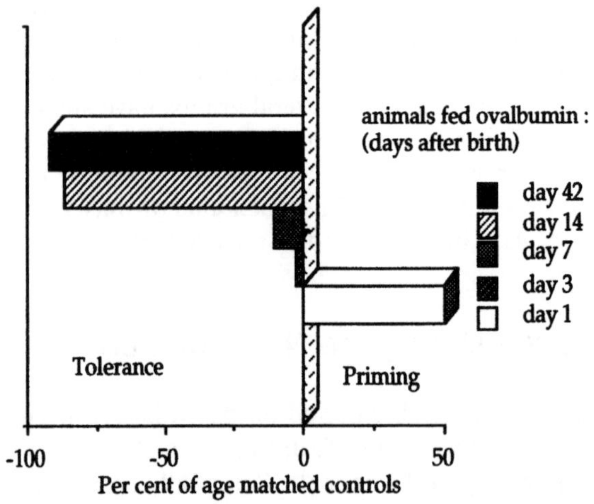

Fig. 3. Age-dependent modulation of oral tolerance to ovalbumin (humoral and cell-mediated immunity). The induction of tolerance for both limbs of the immune response is age dependent. Responses of age-matched controls are taken as 0% change

tomy under general anaesthesia. Controls were injected with either saline or with an unrelated antigen (BSA) (Fig. 4). After the mice were born and normally reared, they were systemically immunised at 28 days of age (following the normal experimental protocol). Significant priming, both for antibody and delayed type hypersensitivity (DTH) responses, was observed in mice "fed" OVA before birth.

Weaning and Modulation of Oral Tolerance to Ovalbumin

Feeding during the weaning period disturbed the normal pattern of tolerance induction. In an experimental design in which the separate effects of age *and* weaning could be examined, animals were fed OVA or saline on the day of weaning and 3 and 7 days before or after weaning. The results are summarised in Fig. 5 and demonstrate that there is a transient reduction of oral tolerance, and that this observation was not age related but the result of the weaning process.

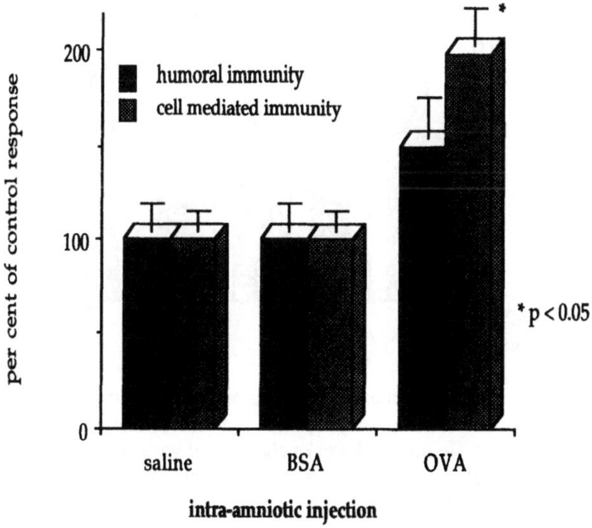

Fig. 4. Effects of prenatal antigen exposure on subsequent immune responses. All animals demonstrate an antigen-specific priming effect after prenatal, enteral antigen exposure. The administration of an unrelated antigen (BSA) does not lead to priming. (All animals immunised with OVA in complete Freund's adjuvant at 4 weeks of age.)

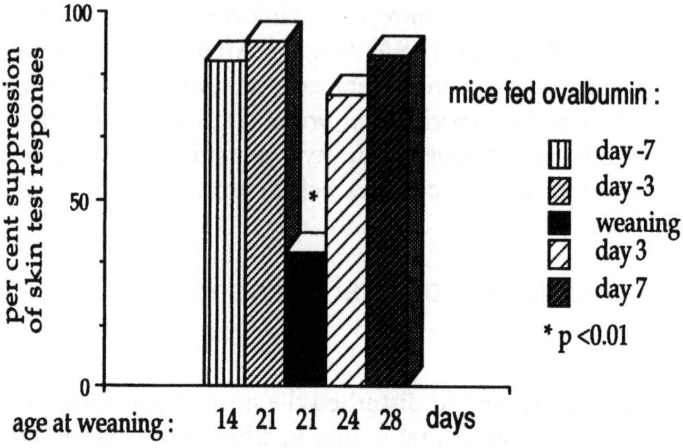

Fig. 5. Transient loss of oral tolerance induction during weaning (cell-mediated immunity). Animals' transient loss of tolerance induction during weaning is not age related but dependent on the day of weaning

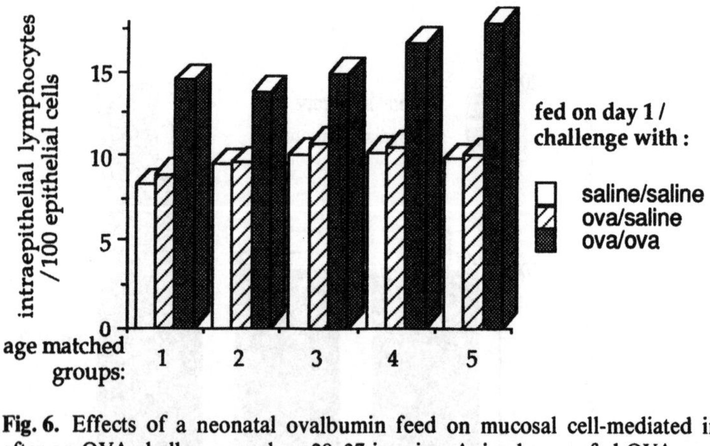

Fig. 6. Effects of a neonatal ovalbumin feed on mucosal cell-mediated immunity after an OVA challenge on days 28–37 in mice. Animals were fed OVA or saline on the 1st day of life and at 4 weeks challenged with OVA for 10 days. Only animals fed OVA and challenged with OVA showed signs of a cell-mediated immune response in the intestinal mucosa

Neonatal Antigen Administration and Induction of Mucosal Cell-Mediated Immunity

Feeding OVA to neonatal animals did not induce a mucosal cell-mediated immune response in the gut. Feeding neonatal animals by gavage at day 1 followed by a challenge in their drinking water at 28 days of age for 10 days led to an increase in intra-epithelial lymphocytes within the jejunal mucosa. This finding suggests induction of mucosal cell-mediated immune response (Fig. 6) [47].

Conclusion

Our knowledge about developmental aspects of food allergy is still scanty and the conclusions drawn from published reports of animal and human studies are sometimes contradictory, if not confusing. It is obvious, however, that immune responses after oral antigen encounter in the neonate (or young infant) are different from adult immune responses, and that they cannot be dissociated from developmental aspects. The final (immunological) outcome after antigen presentation is an equation with a multitude of interrelated variables; these may be summarised as follows:

1. Genetic background (parental history of atopy).
2. Environmental factors (e.g. smoking, pollution).
3. Time of intestinal antigen encounter.
4. Immaturity of digestion (creation of immunochemically different antigen moieties: *tolerogens versus immunogens*?).
5. HLA-DR expression of epithelial cells.
6. Immaturity of gut-associated immune regulation.
7. Effects of breast milk on the neonate's immune system.
8. Neuro-immunological effects of maternal hormones.
9. Age-related differences in macromolecular binding, uptake and mucosal permeability.
10. Immunosuppressive effects of (virus) infections.

Acknowledgements. I would like to thank Prof. ANNE FERGUSON and Dr. ALLAN M. MOWAT for their stimulating and critical discussions during the early experimental work discussed in this paper. The views expressed here are my own. I am also grateful for financial support which was provided by Action Research, the MRC and the Deutsche Forschungsgemeinschaft (STR 210/1-2). I also thank Miss FAITH HANSTATER for skilful preparation of the manuscript.

References

1. Hayward AR (1981) Development of lymphocyte responses and interactions in the human fetus and newborn. Immunol Rev 57:39-60
2. Hill HR (1987) Biochemical, structural, and functional abnormalities of polymorphonuclear leukocytes in the neonate. Pediatr Res 22:375-382
3. Wilson CB (1986) Immunologic basis for increased susceptibility of the neonate to infection. J Pediatr 108:1-12
4. Fietta A, Sacchi F, Bersani C, et al. (1987) Complement-dependent bactericidal activity for E. coli K12 in serum of preterm newborn infants. Acta Paediatr Scand 76:37-41
5. Miyawaki T, Moriya N, Nagaoki T, Taniguchi N (1981) Maturation of B cell differentiation ability and T cell regulatory function in infancy and childhood. Immunol Rev 57:61-88
6. Murgita A, Wigzell H (1981) Regulation of immune functions in the fetus and newborn. Prog Allergy 219:54-113
7. Roberton DM, Paganelli R, Dinwiddie R, Levinsky RJ (1982) Milk antigen absorption in the preterm and term neonate. Arch Dis Child 57:369-372
8. Beach RC, Menzies IS, Clayden GS, Scopes JW (1982) Gastrointestinal permeability changes in the preterm neonate. Arch Dis Child 57:141-145
9. Turner MW, Boulton P, Shields JG, et al. (1987) Uptake of ingested protein from the gut, changes in intestinal permeability to sugars and release of mast cell protease II in rats experiencing locally induced hypersensitivity reactions. In: Chandra RK (ed) Food allergy, St. Johns, Newfoundland, Nutrition Research Foundation, pp 79-94
10. Müller G, Bernsau I, Müller W, Weisbarth-Riedel E, Natzschka J, Rieger CHL (1987) Cow's milk protein antigens and antibodies in the serum of premature infants during the first 10 days of life. J Pediatr 109:869-873
11. Lindberg T, Lothe L, Axelsson I, Benediktsson B (1986) Human alpha-lactalbumin as a marker of macromolecular absorption. Gut 27:1029-34
12. Ehrlich P (1892) Über Immunität durch Vererbung und Säugung, Zeitschr Hygiene und Infektionskrankheiten 12:183-203
13. Ogra SS, Ogra PL (1978) Immunologie aspects of human colostrum and milk. II. Characteristics of lymphocyte reactivity and distribution of E-rosette forming cells at different times after onset of lactation. J Pediatr 92:550-554
14. Hanson L, Ahlstedt S, Andersson B, et al. (1985) Protective factors in milk and the development of the immune system. Pediatrics 75 (suppl.): 172-175
15. Svanborg-Eden C, Carlsson B, Hanson L, et al. (1979) Anti-pili antibodies in breast milk. Lancet 2:1235
16. Kilshaw PJ, Cant AJ (1984) The passage of maternal dietary proteins into human breast milk. Int Arch Allergy Appl Immunol 75:8
17. Gerrard JW (1984) Allergies in breast fed babies to foods ingested by mothers. Clin Rev Allergy 2:143-149

18. Chandra RK, Puri S, Suraiya C, Cheema PS (1986) Influence of maternal food antigen avoidance during pregnancy and lactation on incidence of atopic eczema an infants. Clin Allergy 16:563–569
19. Björksten B (1983) Does breast feeding prevent the development of allergy? Immunol Today 4:215–217
20. Gillin FD, Reiner DS, Wang CS (1983) Human milk kills parasitic intestinal protozoa. Science 221:1290–1291
21. Kramer MS (1988) Does breast feeding help protect against atopic disease - biology, methodology, and a golden jubilee of controversy. J Pediatr 112:182–190
22. Savilhati E, Tainio V-M, Salmenpera L, et al. (1987) Prolonged exclusive breast feeding and heredity as determinants in infantile atopy. Arch Dis Child 62:269–273
23. Dannaeus A, Johannson SGO, Foucard T (1978) Clinical and immunological aspects of food allergy. II. Development of allergic symptoms and humoral immune response to foods in infants of atopic mothers during the first 24 months of life. Acta Paediatr Scand 67:715–718
24. Harmatz PR, Bloch KJ, Kleinman RE, Walsh MK, Walker WA (1986) Influence of circulating maternal antibody on the transfer of dietary antigen to neonatal mice via milk. Immunology 57:43–48
25. Rieger CHL, Kraft SC, Rothberg RM (1980) Lack of effect of passive immunization on the active immune response to an ingested soluble protein antigen. J Immunol 124:1789–1793
26. Müller W, Lippmann A, Rieger CHL (1983) Oral immunization to milk protein in human infants in the presence of passive antibody. Pediatr Res 17:724–728
27. Rothberg RM, Farr RS (1965) Anti bovine serum albumin and anti alpha lactalbumin in the sera of children and adults. Pediatrics 35:381–376
28. Rothberg RM, Rieger CHL, Silverman GA, Peri BA (1981) Antigen uptake and antibody production in the human newborn. In: Orgra PL, Bienenstock J (eds.) First Ross Conference. Ross Laboratories, Columbus 57–62
29. Jarrett EEE (1978) Stimuli for the production and control of IgE in rats. Immunol Rev 41:52–76
30. Jarrett EEE, Hall E (1979) Selective suppression of IgE antibody responsiveness by maternal influence. Nature 280:145–147
31. Jarrett EEE (1984) Perinatal influences on IgE responses. Lancet 2:797–799
32. Mowat AM (1987) The regulation of immune responses to dietary proteins. Immunol Today 8:93–98
33. Strober W (1982) The regulation of mucosal immune system. J Allergy Clin Immunol 70:225–230
34. Strobel S, Mowat AM, Pickering MG, Fersuson A (1983) Immunological responses to fed proteins in mice. 2. Oral tolerance for CMI is due to activation of cyclophosphamide sensitive cells by gut processed antigen. Immunology 49:451–456
35. Vaz N, Maia L, Hanson DG, Lynch J (1977) Inhibition of homocytotropic antibody responses in adult inbred mice by previous feeding of the specific antigen. J Allergy Clin Immunol 60:110–115
36. Korenblatt PE, Rothberg RM, Minden P, Farr PS (1968) Immune responses of human adults after oral and parenteral exposure to bovine serum albumin. J Allergy 41:226–235
37. Lowney ED (1968) Immunologic unresponsiveness to a contact sensitiser in man. J Invest Dermatol 51:411–417

38. Lafont S, André C, Gillon J, Fargier MC (1982) Abrogation by subsequent feeding of antibody response, including IgE in parenterally immunized mice. J. Exp Med 152:1573-1578
39. Strobel S (1984) Modulation of the immune response to fed antigen in mice. Ph.D thesis University of Edinburgh
40. Strobel S, Ferguson A (1987) Persistence of oral tolerance in mice fed ovalbumin is different for humoral and cell mediated immune responses. Immunology 60:317-318
41. Parrott DMV (1976) The gut as a lymphoid organ. Clin Gastroenterol 5:211-228
42. Phillips-Quagliata JM, Roux ME, Amy M, et al. (1983) Migration and regulation of B-cells in the mucosal immune system. Ann NY Acad Sci 409:194-202
43. Strober W, Richman LK, Elson CO (1981) The regulation of the gastrointestinal immune responses. Immunol Today 2:156-162
44. Kilshaw PJ (1981) Gastrointestinal hypersensitivity in the preruminant calf. In: Bourne FJ (ed.) The mucosal immune system. The Hague, Nijhoff 203-219
45. Stokes CR, Newby TJ, Bourne FJ (1983) The influence of oral immunization on local and systemic immune response to heterologous antigens. Clin Exp Immunol 52:399-406
46. Strobel S, Ferguson A (1984) Immune responses to fed antigen in mice. 3. Systemic tolerance or priming is related to age at which antigen is first encountered. Pediatr Res 18:588-594
47. Strobel S, Ferguson A (1986) Modulation of intestinal and systemic immune responses to a fed protein antigen in mice. Gut 27:829-837
48. Stein KE, Söderström T (1984) Neonatal administration of idiotypic or anti-idiotypic antibody primes for protection against *Escherichia coli* K13 infection in mice. J Exp Med 160:1001-1011

The Physiological Humoral Immunologic Response to Alimentary Antigens

C. H. L. Rieger

The gastrointestinal tract represents that part of the organism in which the most intensive interaction between the organism and its environment takes place. Intestinal flora, nutritional antigens, and also most inhaled antigens can be detected in the immunological system of the intestines. Thus, an understanding of immune responses to ingested antigens is required in order to understand pathological immune resposes.

The immune system can react to ingested antigens in four different ways (or a combination thereof):

- The antigen remains undetected.
- A primary specific tolerance occurs.
- An active secretory and/or humoral antibody response takes place, with some physiological significance but without pathologically affecting the individual.
- An excessive immune response occurs which could lead to an allergic reaction.

In the past, the examination of often complicated experimental models has led to the overvaluation of certain kinds of immune responses to oral antigens. CHASE's use of the prior introduction of antigens in the prevention of contact dermatitis led, for example, to the assumption that tolerance induction was the most important result of the use of oral antigens [12]. The observation of physiological active antibody responses to milk proteins in neonates became, on the other hand, falsely associated with allergies. For this reason, it is important to examine the conditions which lead to the different reactions of the immunological system to intestinal antigens.

Under certain circumstances an antigen is not recognized by the immunological system at all. To date, this occurrence has only rarely been examined or has only seldom been taken into consideration, and it seems even to be difficult to simulate. The easiest protocol involves destroying the structure of the antigen. For example, whey proteins in milk can be almost completely denatured through heat exposure, a technique which does not work with casein. Hydrolytic splitting of protein can completely destroy the antigen, and consequently all other qualities of the protein, such as taste, are destroyed as well.

The chemical modification of an antigen should be mentioned as a third possibility. That the conjugation of dodecanyl acid on bovine serum albumin (BSA) and the subsequent ingestion of this antigen led neither to a cellular nor to a humoral response, was readily illustrated by animal experimentation. This missing immunological response was not the result of specific tolerance but, in fact, the result of the antigen not having been recognized. The subsequent injection of the rabbits with pure BSA led to a normal primary response [1]. Although this form of nutritional antigen modification has so far hardly been investigated, it could play an important role in the examination of food allergies.

The second form of immunological responses to oral antigens is immunological tolerance, i.e., the specific deficit of an antibody response to the antigen concerned, sustaining the humoral response towards other antigens. In principle, such a tolerance can in fact be induced, but it results as well when an active humoral response is detectable in advance. Practical experience with primary-induced tolerance seems to have been known for a long time. North American Indians, for example, prevented contact dermatitis from poisonivy (Rhus radicans), by giving their children the plant extract. Since CHASE experimentally obtained a similar effect in mice [12], enormous value has been placed on oral tolerance induction in past decades. Consequently it became possible, for example, to establish long-lasting tolerance by feeding mice only once with small quantities of ovalbumin [2]. If newborn rabbits receive BSA, they resorb large quantities of this protein in an antigenic form. This does not lead to an active humoral response, which is typical in adult rabbits, but to a specific and long-lasting tolerance [3].

Neither the feeding of ivy extracts, the tube feeding with minimal quantities of protein, nor the feeding of foreign protein to newborn rabbits, however, is physiological in action. Observing the tolerance levels in these models should not lead one to the conclusion that this form of immunological response is physiological. The creation of immunological tolerance under physiological conditions is particularly difficult and unusual. It can be produced by feeding an antigen for a very long period of time. With this technique, a decline of specific antibodies to BSA was observed after feeding rabbits for several months. The same phenomenon is known in humans in regard to aging, and despite the continuous absorption of milk proteins the quantity of circulating IgG antibodies to milk proteins diminishes and almost disappears completely when they reach adulthood [4]. This observation is of special interest to pediatricians since existing influences on the immunological system of the mother could possibly determine whether a primary tolerance can be formed in the next generation. In this manner, an immunological tolerance to β-lactoglobulin and α-lactalbumin was established in 8-month-old guinea pigs whose mothers had been fed with appropriate antigens from birth [5]. Yet the outcome of this experiment depended on the continuous feeding of the antigen throughout the entire pregnancy.

The third possible reaction of the immunological system to oral antigens is the active production of circulating and secretory antibodies: this is the physiological manner in which humans and most other mammals react to oral protein. Therefore, understanding this form of immunological response is especially important in the exploration of allergic and other pathologic reactions.

Investigation of the active immunological response to oral antigens starts with examining the antigen itself and observing how it enters the immunological system. Antigenic food proteins can be directly absorbed by the lymphatic tissue of the intestines; that is, they do not need to be absorbed by the blood first. Measuring the resorbed protein antigens in the blood shows that the quantity of such is not directly proportionate to the intensity of the immunological response to intestinal proteins. It seems more likely that a high resorption of antigen proteins induces suppressor T cells in the blood, which regulatively lower the active humoral response. Based on this concept, it can be shown that hyperimmunization resulting in excessive antibody concentrations, which can easily be created parenterally through repeated antigen injections, cannot be incited orally. A diet of large quantities of antigen leads almost immediately to an antibody response, which can be increased by injecting the appropriate antigen, however not by ingesting the antigen, irrespective of the level of concentration. In this way, a decisive and qualitative distinction can be observed with regard to the parenteral form of immunization. In fact, it is amazing how antigens in foodstuffs, in substantially different concentrations, can create an immunological response which falls within a relatively small range. Several years ago it could be proven that the antibody response of neonates to BSA in milk remained constant, even when the concentration of this antigen was reduced ten fold [6]. The concentration of cow's milk proteins in breast milk amounts to only a few nanograms per milliliter, i.e. 4–5 orders of magnitude below that of cow's milk [7]. Nevertheless, these quantities are not only capable of sensitizing but can also lead to the production of IgG anti-β-lactoglobulin or anti-lactalbumin concentrations, which can be compared to the antibody concentrations in cow's milk given to children (Fig. 1).

In addition, the low interference susceptibility of the oral immunological response creates an important contrast to parenteral immunization. While passive antibodies of the latter form of immunization decisively determine the kind and intensity of the immunological response, passive antibodies do not influence the oral immunological response in an infant to a perceptable degree. In this way, it could be demonstrated that the immunological response of infants to BSA – while passive antibodies from the mother were present – was as high as the immunological response of infants who did not have such antibodies [6]. It seems reasonable that the passive protection inherited by the infant from its mother does not hinder the process of active immunization. Compared to this, parenteral immunization, either towards diphtheria toxoid or

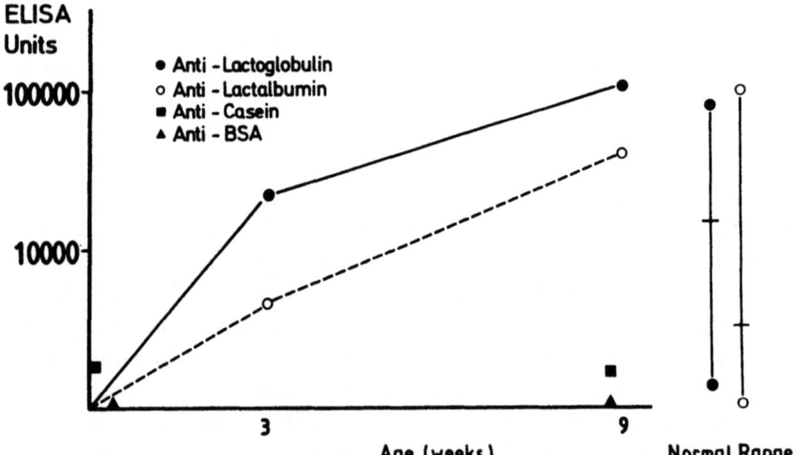

Fig. 1. Milk antibodies in exclusively breast-fed neonate. Serum antibody concentrations at 3 and 9 weeks in an exclusively breast-fed neonate. The figure shows in the normal range a median and a 50% confidence interval of anti-lactoglobuline and anti-lactalbumin in 12 6-month-old neonates fed with cow's milk

measles virus, depends to a critical degree on the intensity of antibody concentration inherited from the mother at the time of injection.

Further characteristics of the physiological immunological response to oral antigens have been examined mainly in connection with cow's milk proteins. Neonates, after the 36th week of gestation, are capable of producing serum antibodies to these proteins within 1–2 weeks. Casein leads to an earlier and more intensive antibody response, however all other cow's milk proteins examined so far have also been identified as being very antigenic. The maximum immunological response to antigens in the serum is reached between 3 and 6 months. Afterwards, an almost constant antibody level exists for serveral years. The antibody concentration to cow's milk proteins diminishes in school-aged children. Only one out of three young adults have antibodies to BSA [4].

To date, only little investigation has been carried out on secretory antibodies to cow's milk proteins. At the end of the 2nd week, ROBERTSON et al. detected secretory IgA to β-lactoglobulin in the breast milk (Hexenmilch) of neonates [8]. For this purpose a special study examined the amount of specific IgA and IgM to β-lactoglobulin and α-casein in the saliva of neonates and detected that specific immunoglobulines of the SIgA and SIgM categories to these antigens are already present in newborn neonates within the first days after birth (Fig. 2). The presence of these antibodies did not depend on their diet. In some neonates they were identified prior to the first feeding. This proves the presence of active antibodies which are induced prenatally and have not been passively obtained [9]. At present it is questionable whether the antigen stimulation that induces these antibodies is created by milk proteins which are transferred into amniotic fluid, or whether another mechanism must be suspected. In any case, the continued production of the secretory antibodies depends on the specific diet. An exclusive diet of mother's milk causes a decrease in secretory cow's milk antibodies in the saliva, whereas a diet of cow's milk has, temporarily, an increasing effect. Near the end of the 1st year, as the quantity of milk in the neonate's diet decreases, the secretory antibodies also decrease.

The immunological reaction of premature infants to milk proteins is notably different. During the first weeks of their lives, prematurely born infants absorb more β-lactoglubin, in contrast to mature infants who absorb much less casein [10]. Against both antigens, circulating antibodies appear in lower concentrations than with mature infants. This effect can be detected even after 4 weeks, and after 6 month in the case of BSA [11]. Similar to newborn rabbits, human infants seem to form a specific and enduring tolerance to some digestable proteins.

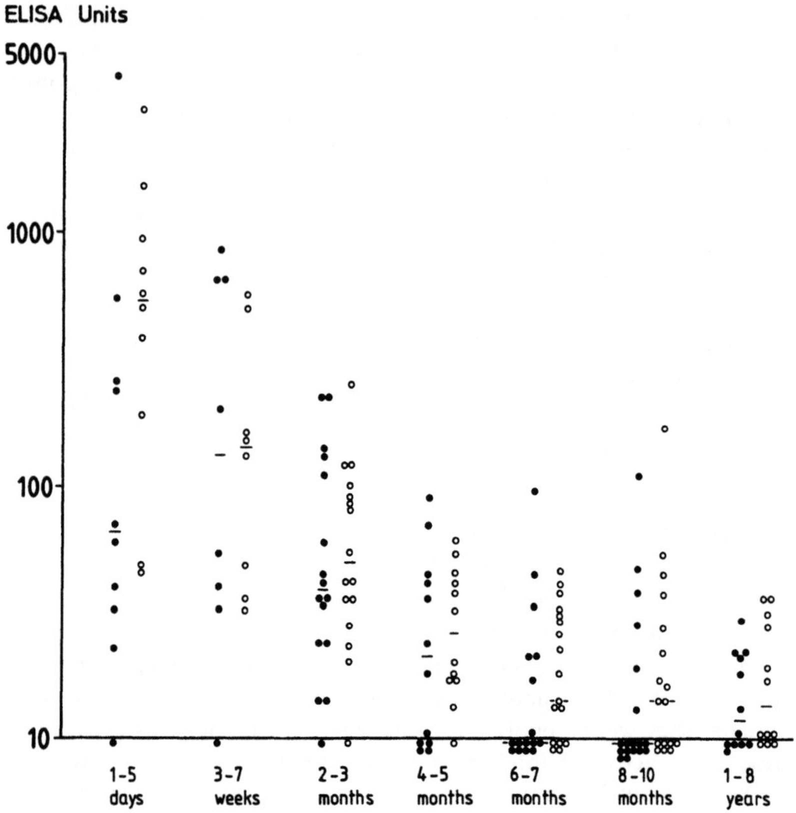

Fig. 2. Antibodies to α-casein in the saliva of healthy children ranging in age from 1 day to 8 years old. *Closed circles* represent the values of IgA antibodies; *open circles*, the values of all antibodies that carry a secretory piece (SIgA or SIgM). (From [9])

The fourth possible immunological response to oral antigens is an exaggerated immunological reaction, leading to clinical symptoms and signs of allergy. However, the production of excessive amounts of antibodies to counteract digestible proteins, e.g., cow's milk proteins, does not necessarily produce allergic reactions. The repeated aspiration of milk, for example, can also result in a substantially higher immune response without inducing clinical symptoms. The mere fact of a higher humoral immunological response should not necessarily be regarded as having pathological significance.

Finally, the immunological response to a particular antigen can be characterized by its qualitative change during the entire feeding process. When guinea pigs are fed ovalbumin for a period of 2 weeks, subsequent inhalation of this antigen can produce bronchial spasms. This reaction ceases to occur on continuation of feeding and in spite of the persistance of specific IgG antibody, possibly because concentrations of the critical asthma-causing antibody. IgG1 anti-ovalbumin, decrease.

In summary, one can conclude the following:

- The oral immunological response is qualitatively and quantitatively different from the imunological response to parenteral antigens.
- The active secretory and serum antibody formation respresents the physiological response to most antigens.
- The oral immunological response bears no direct relationship to the quantity or concentration of antigens, even in instances of high concentration.
- Passive antibodies influence the immunological response only slightly, if at all.
- The continuous ingestion of antigens can result in a modification of the immunological response, so that either total IgG antibody or a IgG-subclass specific antibody is reduced.
- The oral immunological response is induced by the direct penetration of the antigen into the lymphatic tissue of the intestines and is disproportionate to the concentration of the circulating antigen.

In spite of the fact that most of these principles are universally accepted, different conclusions may be drawn under different laboratory conditions. In particular, the application of work conducted on animals to the immune system of man is difficult and should be done with extreme caution.

References

1. Lustig JV, Rieger CHL, Kraft SC, Hunter R, Rothberg RM (1976) Humoral and cellular responses to native antigen following oral and parenteral immunization with lipid-conjugated bovine serum albumin. Cell Immunol 24:164–172
2. Miller SD, Hanson DG (1979) Inhibition of specific immune response by feeding protein antigen. J Immunol 123:2344–2349
3. Rieger CHL, Gülden P, Byrd DJ (1981) Induction of specific tolerance to ingested soluble protein in neonatal rabbits. Immunobiology 160:330–339
4. Korenblat PE, Rothberg RM, Mindern P, Farr RS (1968) Immune responses of human adults after oral and parenteral exposure to bovine serum albumin. Journal of Allergy 41:226–235
5. Telemo E, Jakobson J, Weström BR, Folkesson H (1987) Maternal dietary antigens and the immune response in the offspring of the guinea pig. Immunology 62:35–38
6. Müller W, Lippmann A, Rieger CHL (1983) Oral immunization to milk protein in human infants in the presence of passive antibody. Pediatr Res 17:724–728
7. Kilshaw PJ, Lant AJ (1984) The passage of maternal dietary proteins into human breast milk. Int Arch Allergy Appl Immunol 75:8–15
8. Robertson DM, Forrest PJ, Frangonlis E, Jones CL Mermelstein N (1986) Early induction of secretory immunity in infancy: specific antibody in neonatal breast milk. Arch Dis Child 61:489–494
9. Frick M, Rieger CHL (1987) Local antibodies to α-casein and β-lactoglobulin in the saliva of infants. Pediatr Res 22:399–401
10. Müller G, Bernsau I, Müller W, Weissbarth-Riedel E, Natzschka J, Rieger CHL (1986) Cow milk protein antigens and antibodies in serum of premature infants during the first 10 days of life. J Pediatr 109: 869–873
11. Helms, Rieger CHL (1987) Decreased production of specific antibodies to cow's milk proteins in premature infants during the first six months of life. Eur J Pediatr 146:131–134
12. Chase MW (1946) Inhibition of experimental drug allergy by prior feeding of the sensitizing agent. Proc Soc Exp Biol Med 61:257–259

Food Antigens in Human Milk

I. Jakobsson

Today we know, mostly from animal experiments, that macromolecules, like food antigens, can pass through the intestinal barrier into the circulation. The molecules can reach the mother's milk and also pass the placental barrier to reach to foetus. In recent years we have also obtained evidence that this macromolecular transport takes place in humans. In 1921 SHANNON [1] described breast-fed infants with eczema and one infant with colic and diarrhoea. All the infants showed intolerances to foods that they had never eaten. These reactions were mostly against egg white. The mothers were told to eat no foods containing eggs, and the eczema disappeared, but returned again when the mothers once more ate eggs. To verify his hypothesis that egg white eaten by the mother could pass into her milk, SHANNON also carried out anaphylactic experiments on the milk given to guinea pigs. From 1930 and to the present there has been rather little written about this phenomenon.

Today, with the trend towards increased breast feeding, there is also an increasing interest in studying manifestations of food intolerances in totally breast-fed infants.

About 10 years ago we started a study in infants with cow's milk protein intolerance. We found that many infants with this intolerance had colic as one symptom. We also found that before being diagnosed as cow's milk protein intolerant, many infants had already suffered from substantial feeding difficulties when fed only human milk. This led us to the hypothesis that cow's milk taken by the mother can reach the infant via the breast milk. We have since tested this hypothesis on a number of infants with infantile colic [2, 3]. In the first series, 12/19 were symptom free when their mothers pursued a diet free of cow's milk proteins, but upon increasing the size of the series we could conclude that about one-third of breast-fed infants with infantile colic remain free of symptoms when their mothers are on a cow's milk free diet.

We have also developed a radioimmunological method to analyse the content of cow's milk proteins in human milk, measuring the bovine protein β-lactoglobulin [4]. Figure 1 shows the results of repeated analyses of human milk from three mothers beginning a cow's milk free diet. During these first few days, the content of β-lactoglobulin decreased and the symptoms of colic in their infants disappeared. Figure 2 reports the effects of giving one glass of cow's milk to one mother treated with a cow's milk free diet. The content of bovine β-lactoglobulin in the human milk increased and reached a maximum after 8–12 h.

We have also followed a group of mothers during their entire lactation period. Milk samples were collected every 2nd week [5]. We recorded family history of allergy, the mother's intake of cow's milk, and existing symptoms in the infants. A total of 232 milk samples from 25 mothers were analysed (Fig. 3). The content of β-lactoglobulin varied greatly between samples from one mother to another and also between samples from the same mother. All mothers had a diet containing a

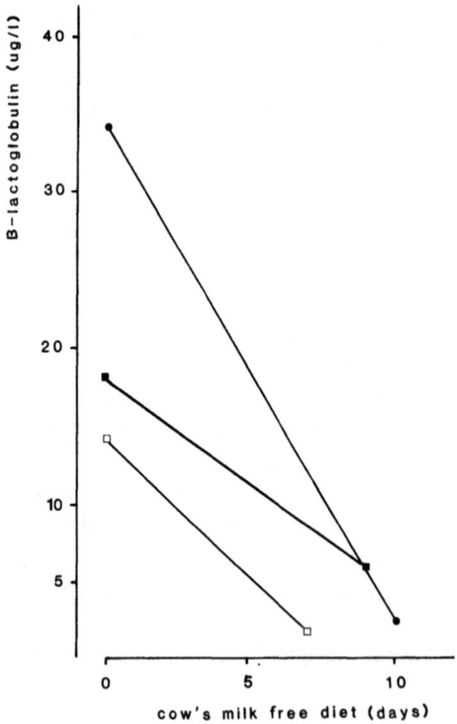

Fig. 1. Influence of a cow's milk free diet on the content of β-lactoglobulin in the human milk from three mothers with colicky infants

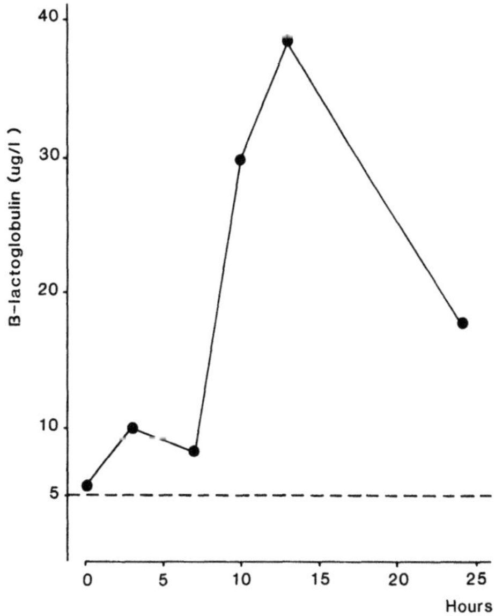

Fig. 2. Content of β-lactoglobulin in the breast milk of one mother after drinking 250 ml cow's milk (at time 0 h)

quantity of cow's milk of between 200 and 1500 ml per day. β-Lactoglobulin was detected in 93/232 milk samples (40%). Six mothers had no detectable β-lactoglobulin on any occasion. Two mothers (indicated in the figure) had measurable β-lactoglobulin in all their milk samples. There was no difference in intake of cow's milk between the six mothers without β-lactoglobulin and the two with β-lactoglobulin in all samples. Seven mothers had more than 50 μg/l β-lactoglobulin in at least one milk sample. In six of their infants there were complaints of diarrhoea, vomiting or exanthemas. Of the 18 mothers with a β-lactoglobulin content of less than 50 μg/l the same symptoms occurred in five infants. This difference is statistically significant. We found no correlation between history of allergy and content of β-lactoglobulin in the breast milk. However, the one mother with a high concentration of β-lactoglobulin in all her milk samples had a pronounced family history of allergy. The wide variation in content of β-lactoglobulin between different mothers could have serveral explanations. Different mothers may have different concentrations of secretory IgA antibodies to β-lactoglobulin in their milk. Serum antibodies to β-lactoglobulin in the mothers may be of importance.

Other invesigators have also shown a content of food antigens in the human milk. STUART et al. [6] measured the content of β-lactoglobulin

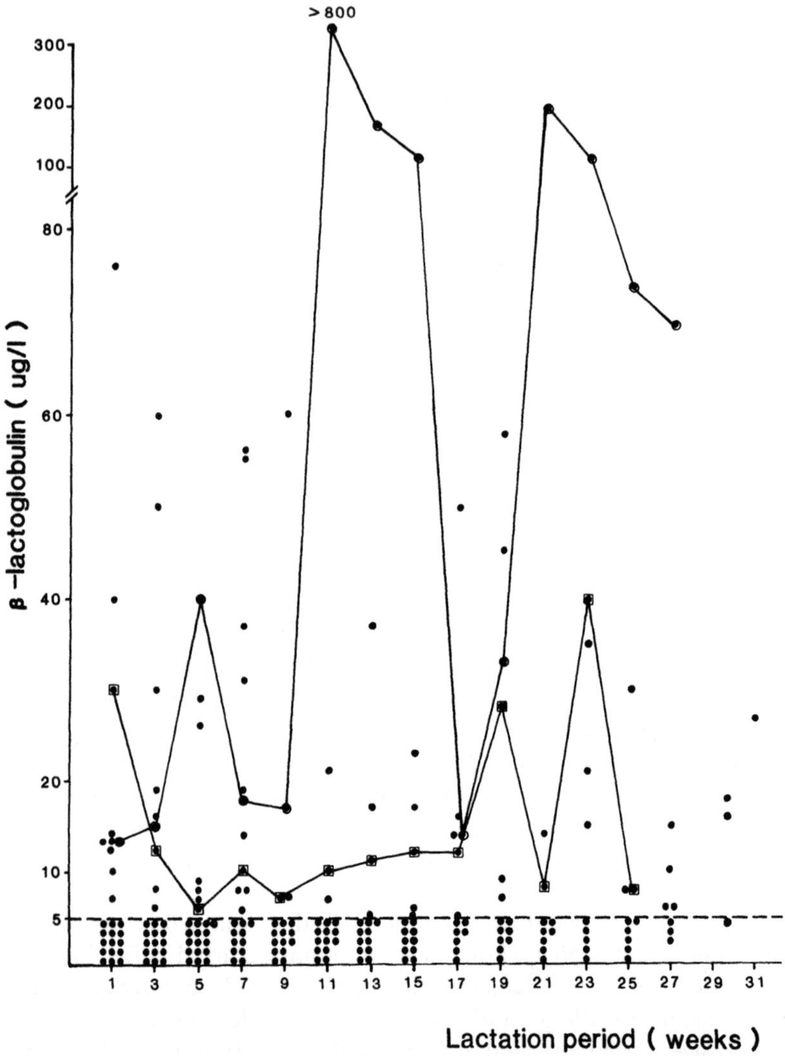

Fig. 3. Content of β-lactoglobulin (μg/l) in 232 human milk samples from 25 mothers. (Values below 5 μg/l were not measurable.) □—□, ○—○, Two mothers with detectable amounts in all milk samples

with an enzyme-linked immunosorbent assay (ELISA) technique and found that 18% (compared to our 40%) of mothers had detectable levels of β-lactoglobulin in their milk. CANT et al. [7] studied the relationship between cow's milk or egg proteins in human milk and eczema in infants. They found concentrations of ovalbumin in the milk of the same magnitude both in mothers with and in those without infants with eczema. This illustrates one aspect of the problem of food antigens in human milk – the risk of sensitization and development of food allergy already when fed only breast milk. This is perhaps only a minor problem as the development of intolerance may be the exeption rather than the rule.

I would now like to discuss a further aspect of this phenomenon. The content of food antigens in human milk may be of importance for development of a proper immunological response to common food antigens in the very young infant, i.e. a development of tolerance.

I have carried out work in animals in collaboration with zoophysiologists [8, 9]. It is quite clear in studies of the rat that heterologous macromolecules emanating from the food of the mother can reach the foetus and the suckling offspring of the mother. From a physiological point of view, it is tempting to speculate that the existence of food antigens both in foetal circulation and in mother's milk is a naturally occurring event for the common proteins in normal food. In mice it has been shown [10] that intraperitoneal injection of human γ-globulins to lactating mice results in systemic tolerance in the nursing offspring, specific to these proteins. It has also been shown that the specific protein content in the diet of the pregnant and lactating rabbit [11] is of importance for the immunological response of the offspring; the offspring becomes immunologically tolerant to proteins included in the mother's diet.

In a study that we conducted [12], a group of female guinea pigs were fed a diet containing cow's milk protein from early in life. These females were then mated, and the diet of their offspring were varied regarding cow's milk protein. At 3 months of age all second-generation animals were challenged by an intraperitoneal injection of cow's milk protein, and immune responses were studied as serum IgG and a tracheal Schultz-Dale response to cow's milk protein. All guinea pigs born to mothers fed cow's milk showed a reduced immune response compared to controls born to mothers fed a cow's milk free diet. The results showed that by including protein antigens in the mothers' diet it was possible to alter the immune response to these antigens in the offspring, despite the lack of direct contact between offspring and antigen before the challenge.

We know from studies in both animals and humans that food antigens can reach the foetus or the newborn breast-fed infant or animal via the mother. This is probably a naturally occurring phenomenon that may be of importance in the development of a proper immunological response to common food antigens, however it may also be of importance in causing a sensitization and a development of food allergy in infants with an allergic predisposition.

References

1. Shannon WR (1921) Demonstration of food proteins in human breast milk by anaphylactic experiments on guinea pigs. Am J Dis Child 22:2223–2231
2. Jakobsson I, Lindberg T (1979) Cow's milk as a cause of infantile colic in breast fed infants. Lancet II:437–439
3. Jakobsson I, Lindberg T (1983) Cow's milk proteins cause infantile colic in breast fed infants: a double-blind crossover study. Pediatrics 71:268–271
4. Jakobsson I, Lindberg T, Benediktsson B, Hansson BG (1985) Dietary bovine β-lactoglobulin is transferred to human milk. Acta Paediatr Scand 74:342–345
5. Axelsson I, Jakobsson I, Lindberg T, Benediktsson B (1986) Bovine β-lactoglobulin in the human milk. A longitudinal study during the whole lactation period. Acta Paediatr Scand 75:702–707
6. Stuart CA, Twiselton R, Nicholas MK, Hide DW (1984) Passage of cow's milk protein in breast milk. Clin Allergy 14:533–535
7. Cant A, Marsden RA, Kilshaw PJ (1985) Egg and cow's milk hypersensitivity in exclusively breast fed infants with eczema and detection of egg protein in breast milk. Br Med J 291:932–935
8. Dahl GMK, Telemo E, Weström BR, Jakobsson I, Lindberg T, Karlsson BW (1984) The passage of orally fed proteins from mothers to foetus in the rat. Comp Biochem Physiol [A] 77A:199–201
9. Telemo E, Weström B, Dahl G, Karlsson B (1986) Transfer of orally or intravenously administered proteins to the milk of the lactating rat. J Pediatr Gastroenterol Nutr 5:305–309
10. Halsey JF, Benjamin DC (1976) Induction of immunologic tolerance in nursing neonates by absorption of tolerogen from colostrum. J Immunol 116:1204–1207
11. Pathriana C, Goulding NJ, Gibney MJ, Jennifer M, Gallagher PJ, Taylor TG (1981) Immune tolerance produced by pre- and postnatal exposure to dietary antigens. Int Arch Allergy Appl Immunol 66:114–118
12. Telemo E, Jakobsson I, Weström BR, Folkesson H (1987) Maternal dietary antigens and the immune response in the offspring of the guinea pig. Immunology 62:35–38

Pseudo-Allergic Reactions to Food

D. A. Moneret-Vautrin and Y. Maria

The concept of pseudo-allergic reactions to food, or false food allergies (FFA) has now gained wide acceptance [1–3]. Disregarding food toxicity and intolerance related to enzyme deficiencies, FFA were first defined as clinical reactions to food which mimic allergic reactions but lack immunological mechanisms. More recently it has become possible to diagnose food allergy by two series of tests: (a) skin and laboratory tests that show evidence of specific IgE and (b) single- or double-blind provocation tests that confirm the involvement of these antibodies in the pathology under investigation [4–6].

Having thus defined the immediate type of food allergy (and ignoring the possibility of some cases of food allergies induced by other mechanisms), non-immunological adverse reactions are easier diagnosed. A study reporting 230 cases of FFA listed the main symptoms as: chronic urticaria or recurrent Quincke's oedema (75%), defects of intestinal function (40%), vasomotor headaches (16.8%), rhinitis (10.8%), asthma (5.6%), anaphylactoid shock (1.7%), exacerbation of atopic dermatitis, and psychological symptoms [6].

It is difficult to estimate the prevalence of food intolerance in the general population. Food allergy may be present in 1%–3% of adults and in three times as many children. FFA seems to be three to five times more frequent, both in children, who often eat much histamine-releasing food (e.g. strawberries and chocolate) and food colourings, and in adults, who may have a diet imbalance in favour of food rich in histamine or tyramine (e.g. fermented cheese, sausage and alcohol). According to MAY and BOCK [8], food allergy is encountered in only one-third of the subjects who show an intolerance and, according to BOCK [7] in only 20% of children.

Three major mechanisms are involved in FFA [9]:

1. An abnormal intake of biogenic amines, such as histamine, tyramine and phenylethylamine.

2. An abnormal release of chemical mediators from mast cells. The histaminic mechanism is well identified, but other mediators issuing from arachidonic acid may play a role. Skin mast cells seem to be prone to histamine-releasing agents, but the location of histamine release in the gut, from the mucosal mast cells, is postulated.
3. Interference by food or additives with the autonomic system.

The fascinating concept of immunotoxicity, which is currently used for xenobiotics such as drugs and chemical substances, may be enlarged to include food and food additives. Immunotoxicity includes immune deficiency, autoimmune disorders, carcinogenicity and hypersensitivity. Except for immune deficiency, good examples of autoimmune disorders, carcinogenicity and hypersensitivity induced by food may be provided – such as rheumatoid polyarthritis induced by an allergy to milk proteins or aflatoxin-induced carcinogenicity.

Regarding exclusively hypersensitivity, several theoretically distinct types of FFA accord with different levels of the sequence (Fig. 1). These include (a) harmful stimuli, at the membrane level, of mast cells, basophils, platelets, lymphocytes or other cells and (b) exogenous intake of the chemical mediator histamine. An intriguing alternative may

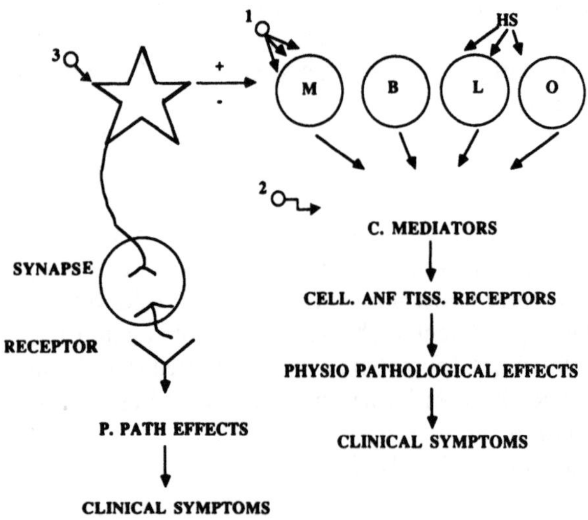

Fig. 1. Hypersensitivity (*HS*) and pseudo-allergic reactions. *1*, Non-specific membrane stimulation; *2*, exogenous intake of biogenic amines; *3*, interference of food and chemicals with neurons, neurotransmitters and neuroreceptors. *M*, mast cells; *B*, basophils; *L*, lymphocytes; *O*, other cells

be the absence of intake of normal precursors of chemical mediators; recent studies seem to indicate that patients with atopic dermatitis have an enzyme deficiency which could impair the synthesis of arachidonic acid by lowering the level of precursors. In some patients this hypothesis is supported by the plasma profiles of essential fatty acids (EFA). Patients who ingest evening primrose oil containing the precursor γ-linolenic acid have been seen to improve. If this finding is confirmed, atopic dermatitis may be considered a partially non-immunological reaction, mediated by the absence of intake in a sufficient amount of normal precursors [10]. Defective EFA metabolism may contribute to T-lymphocyte abnormalities.

These theoretical sites of interaction between food components, cells and mediators would fit clinical symptoms mimicking allergic ones: anaphylactoid shock, intrinsic asthma, nasal polyposis, chronic urticaria, recurrent Quincke's oedema, perennial rhinitis, digestive disorders with diarrhoea, and abdominal pain. It could be postulated that different abnormalities preclude these forms of FFA. The abnormalities may be related to the releasibility of the cells or to the receptivity of receptors to chemical mediators. The fact that an atopic background is often observed in patients with FFA to food would be in keeping with this hypothesis since an abnormal releasibility of basophils has been observed in different subsets of atopic patients [11].

On the other hand, we must not neglect the importance of the autonomic nervous system (ANS), the possible involvement of which in FFA must be underlined. First, the immune modulation by neurotransmitters such as substance P, somatostatin and encephalin may play a role [12] (Fig. 1). Second, clinical symptoms may proceed from abnormal influx of the ANS. This abnormal reactive state of the ANS may be evoked either by caffein and thein, stimulating adrenergic receptors and

Table 1. The role of atopic background in false food allergy

	Food allergy ($n = 130$)	False food allergy ($n = 245$)
Previous history of eczema or asthma	63%	45%
Positive skin tests to common allergens	66%	25%
Increased total IgE levels		
Adults	46.5%	18%
Children <8 years old	83%	70%

sodium metabisulphites, triggering a vagal reflex and eliciting a cholinergic-induced asthma; by other food additives interfering with the dopaminergic and cholinergic transmission, such as erythrosin B [13], or with the serotoninergic and adrenergic transmission, in experimental models using BHT or BHA; or by monosodium glutamate, enhancing the synthesis of acetylcholine [9]. In the context of clinical reactions that proceed by food-induced stimulation of the ANS, one can consider vasomotor rhinitis, the irritable bowel syndrome, the hyperreactive child syndrome and the hyperventilation syndrome.

In current practice, adverse reactions with histamine-rich foods are well characterized. An excessive intake is not sufficient to elicit reactions, since protective mechanisms toward exogenous histamine exist at the intestinal and at the hepatic level. At the intestinal level, mucoproteins in the intestinal lumen can bind some histamine, the rest passes into the mucosa and is subjected to enzymatic degradation by amine oxidases or undergoes phagocytosis by the eosinophils. At the hepatic level, histamine transmitted through the portal vein may be degraded by hepatic methyltransferase, the synthesis of which is impaired in the case of viral hepatitis [14–16].

A study on volunteers undergoing cholecystectomy showed that portal histamine remained stable when 72 mg histamine was instilled into the duodenum. When more than 102 mg was instilled, a raised portal histamineaemia was observed, but the liver maintained a normal posthepatic level; this was the case even with 180 mg [17]. When 1.75 mg/kg histamine was instilled into the duodenum of controls, there was only a slight tachycardia and a facial flush lasting no more than 5 min. The same symptoms were observed in three patients with coeliac disease. In 60% of patients with FFA, however, pruritis, flush, and sometimes tachycardia urticaria or vasomotor headaches were noted, lasting 10–30 min. More recently plasmatic histamine was evaluated before and at 5, 15 and 45 min after the instillation in patients with chronic urticaria and FFA. In 20% of patients there was an increased histaminaemia at 5 min, reflecting an abnormal mucosal permeability. Some maintained a high level at 15 and 45 min, indicating an impaired catabolism. Enzymatic dysfunctions of monoamine oxydases or of hepatic methyltransferase must be postulated. There was no significant correlation between increased levels of plasmatic histamine and clinical symptoms. This result leads us to believe that chronic urticaria with FFA is mainly due to an abnormal receptivity of receptors to histamine.

The second frequent type of FFA to food is related to histamine-releasing foods, such as ovomucoid from egg white, crustaceans, strawberries, tomatoes, fish, pork, chocolate and alcohol. According to De Weck, pineapple and papaya, which contain proteolytic enzymes, and leguminous plants and peanuts, which contain lectins, may also be involved, as well as bacterial endotoxins or fungal substances that lead to the formation of anaphylatoxins [2]. The predominant site for non-specific histamine release is the skin mast cells [18]. In most cases, the affected children have Quincke's oedema or urticaria upon eating strawberries or chocolate. But local degranulation of gut mucosal mast cells (MMC) must be considered by the clinician since the same children often complain simultaneously of abdominal pain. This point is controversial. Indeed, the MMC are numerous in the lamina propria, numbering some 20000 per cubic millimeter [19]. Isolated MMC have been demonstrated to be unresponsive to compound 48/80, bee venom peptide 401 and other histamine releasing agents such as formyl-methionine peptide [20]. Our current knowledge about MMC derives from experimental studies on isolated cells from biopsies obtained by gut surgery. It does not take into account possible abnormalities in patients with FFA, such as cellular magnesium deficiency, which is observed in 45% of patients [6]. In animals, magnesium deficiency increases the releasibility of skin mast cells [21]. We studied biopsies of duodenal mucosa in patients with FFA and observed various ultrastructural aspects of degranulation; however, in biopsies from controls, mast cells were normally granulated [22].

The crucial role of the epithelial and axonal environment of the MMC has to be pointed to (Fig. 2): epithelial irritants such as alcohol, spices and aspirin may create axon reflexes through amyelinic fibres, thus liberating neuropeptides such as substance P which can provoke histamine release from mast cells. This creates the conditions of local hyperpermeability of the epithelium and the small subepithelial vessels, allowing an increased passage of food proteins and additives, and this in turn may enhance FFA and food allergy, which are then interrelated.

Increasing attention is being paid to food additives. Systematic challenges in patients with asthma, urticaria, atopic dermatitis, rhinitis and nasal polyposis show that these are frequently implicated [23–27]. Understanding hypersensivity and non-immunological mechanisms here confronts a landscape which is variable with each specific additive. Nickel salts, which may frequently be implicated in exacerbation of atopic dermatitis, act as haptens, whereas sodium metabisulfites, which elicit severe crises of asthma in 2%–10% of patients with asthma, act as irritants for the bronchial epithelium, triggering a vagal reflex [28]. Moreover, pharmacological or toxic effects of additives may worsen

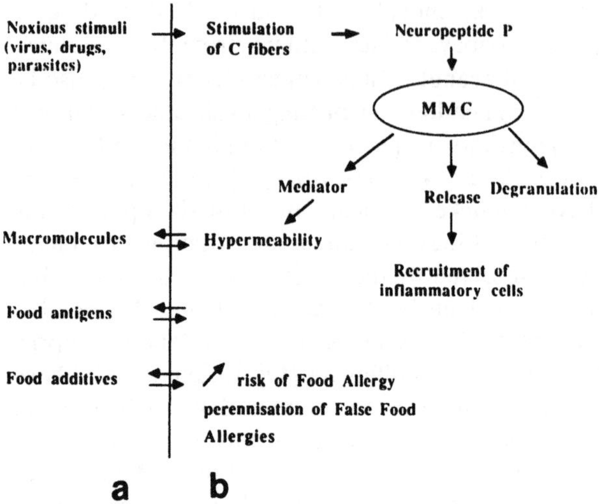

Fig. 2. Modulation of immunological and pharmacological reactions in the gut. *a*, lumen; *b*, mucosa; *MMC*, mucosal mast cells

other types of FFA by inhibiting enzymes such as sodium nitritis, which inhibits monoamine oxydases, or by irritating the mucosa, such as in the case of carragenan.

Finally, establishing the appropriate diagnosis schedule is a complex problem with FFA. That which we currently use is presented in Fig. 3.

Not only are pharmacological actions of food components involved but also the functional state of the digestive mucosa and often a peculiar hyperreactivity to histamine. Various factors play a role. The intake of aspirin or other drugs as well as intestinal fungal infestation may alter the normal functional state of the gut mucosa. Cellular magnesium deficiency and a hyperadrenergic state may favour the hyperreactivity to histamine. Diet imbalance is the key to clinical reactions. As all of these abnormalities can be avoided or suppressed, the diagnosis of FFA would be a satisfying one for the patient, for it implies that he will be cured. Great care is required in management of the diagnosis schedule, and physicians need complete labelling of the offending food. Challenges are obligatory to confirm the usefulness of avoiding the offending food or food additives.

In all cases, fully explained and appropriate instructions should be provided to the patient in order to encourage proper therapeutic observance.

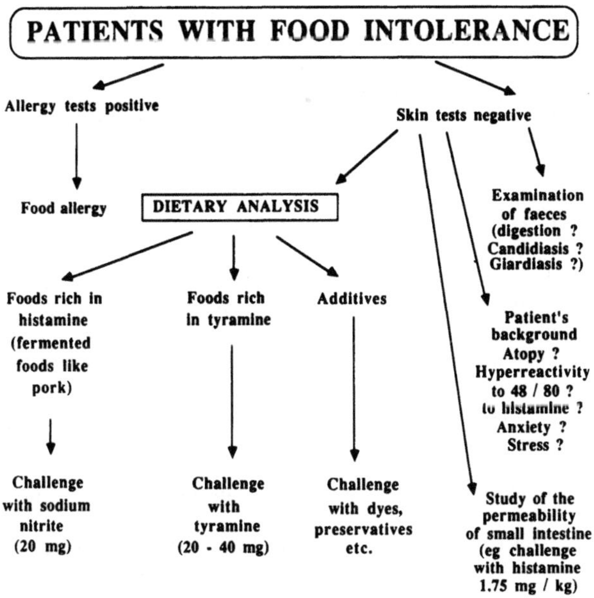

Fig. 3. The diagnosis of false food allergy

References

1. Atkins FM, Metcalf DD (1984) The diagnosis and treatment of food allergy. Annu Rev Nutr 4:233–255
2. De Weck AL (1984) Pathophysiologic mechanisms of allergic and pseudo-allergic reactions to foods, food additives and drugs. Ann Allergy 53:583–586
3. Moneret-Vautrin DA (1983) False food allergies: non-specific reation to foodstuffs. In: Lessof MH (ed) Clinical reactions to food. Wiley, Chichester, pp 135–153
4. Atkins FM, Steinberg SS, Metcalf DD (1985) Evaluation of immediate adverse reactions to foods in adult patients. II. A detailed analysis of reaction patterns during oral food challenge. J Allergy Immunol 75:356–363
5. Bock SA, Lee WY, Remigio LK, May CD (1978) Studies of hypersensitivity reactions to food in infants and children. J Allergy Clin Immunul 62:327–334
6. Moneret-Vautrin DA, Andre Cl (1983) Immunopathologie de l'allergie alimentaire et fausses allergies alimentaires. Masson, Paris, p 266
7. Bock SA (1986) The natural history of adverse reactions to foods. New Engl Reg Allergy Proe 7:504–510
8. May CD, Bock SA (1978) Adverse reactions to food due to hypersensivity. In: Middleton E, Reed CE, Ellis EF (eds) Allergy, principles and practice. Mosby, St Louis, pp 1159–1171

9. Moneret-Vautrin DA (1987) Food intolerance masquerading as food allergy: false food allergy. In: Brostoff J, Challacombe SJ (eds) Food allergy and intolerance. Baillière Tindall, London, pp 836-849
10. Wright S (1985) Atopic dermatitis and essential fatty acids: a biochemical basis for atopy? Acta Derm Venereol 114 (Suppl.): 143-145
11. Butler JM, Ebertz M, Chan SC, Stevens SR, Sobieszczuk D, Hanifin JM (1985) Basophil histamine release in atopic dermatitis and it relationship to disordered cyclic nucleotide metabolism. Acta Derm Venereol 114:55-60
12. Goetzl EJ, Chernou T, Renold F, Payan D (1985) Neuropeptide relation of the expression of immediate hypersensitivity. J Immunol 135:805
13. Augustine JG, Levitan H (1980) Neuro-transmitter release from a vertebrate neuro-muscular synapse affected by a food dye. Science 207:1489-1490
14. Kusche J, Lorentz W (1975) Oxidative deamination of biogenic amines by intestinal amine oxidases: histamine is specifically inactivated by diamine oxidase. Hoppe Seylers Z Physiol Chem: 1485-1496
15. Lindhall KM (1960) The histamine methylating enzyme system in liver. Acta Physiol Scand 22:964-970
16. Marley E, Thomas DV (1976) Histamine and its metabolites in cat portal venous blood and intestine after duodenal instillation of histamine J. Physiol. 263:273 P-274 P
17. Moneret-Vautrin DA, Viniaker J et al (1981) Effets de l'instillation d'histamine dans l'intestin grêle chez l'homme. I. Variation de l'histaminémie portale et périphérique. Ann Gastroentérol Hepatol 17:395-400
18. Juhlin L (1967) Localization and content of histamine in normal and diseased skin. Acta Dermatol 47:383-391
19. Fox CC, Dvorak AM, Peters SP (1985) Isolation and characterization of human intestinal mucosal mast cells. J Immunol 135:483-491
20. Pearce FL, Befus AD, Gauldie J, Bienenstock J (1982) Mucosal mast cells. II. Effects of anti-allergic compounds on histamine secretion by isolated intestinal mast cells. J Immunol 128:2481-2486
21. Bois P (1963) Effect of magnesium deficiency on mast cells and urinary histamine in rats. Br J Exp Pathol 44:151-155
22. Moneret-Vautrin DA, De Korwin JD, Tisserant J (1984) Ultrastructural study of the mast cells of the human duodenal mucosa. Clin Allergy 14:471-479
23. Freedman BJ (1977) Asthma induced by sulfur dioxide, benzoate and tartrazine contained in orange drinks. Clin Allergy 7:407-415
24. Ortolani C., Pastorello E, Luraghi MR et al (1984) Diagnosis of intolerance to food additives. Ann Allergy 53:587-591
25. Supramaniam G, Warner JO (1986) Artificial food additive intolerance in patients with angio-oedema and urticaria. Lancet 18:907-909
26. Benton EC, Barnetson RC (1985) Skin reactions to foods in patients with atopic dermatitis. Acta Derm Venereol 114 (Suppl): 129-132
27. Moneret-Vautrin DA (1986) Tests de provocation aux médicaments, additifs et aliments: recherche d'une hypersensibilité et d'une intolérance. In: Immunologie et Allergie en DRL. Wayoff M, Freche C (eds), Arnette, Paris, pp 201-204
28. Stevenson DD, Simon RA (1981) Sensitivity to ingested metabisulfites in asthmatic subjects. J Allergy Clin Immunol 68:26-32

Clinical Recognition of the Child with Food Allergy

D. J. Hill

The multiplicity of poorly defined illnesses and the variability of pathological lesions induced by various foods in sensitized children have led to a reluctance to recognize various forms of food allergy and to confusion with other forms of food intolerance. Many paediatricians have become increasingly sceptical of various clinical illnesses attributed to food allergy due to evidence that many adults with such illnesses suffer from psychiatric disorders [1] and to the recent recognition that restriction of food intake in childhood, incorrectly attributed to food allergy, constitutes a concealed form of child abuse [2]. In this discussion, food allergy is defined as an adverse reaction to a food substance which is attributed to an immunological hypersensitivity. This concept implies an interaction between one or more food antigens with one or more immune mechanisms leading to the adverse clinical response. Thus, the following discussions confined to IgE-associated conditions, and the terms food allergy and food-protein intolerance are used interchangeably.

The nature of allergic reactions to all foods commonly ingested in childhood has not been studied in detail. However, cow's milk allergy (CMA) has been the subject of intense clinical and laboratory investigation. In this discussion, CMA is used as a model of food allergy in order to appreciate the potential range of manifestations of childhood food allergy which is encountered in clinical practice. These observations are related here to patterns of clinical reactions seen in children with allergic responses to some other common foods.

Common Clinical Syndromes Associated with CMA

CMA affects 2% of infants [3], although incidences of up to 7.5% have been reported [4]. There is evidence of specific humoral [5–7] and cellular [8] immune mechanisms in the CMA reaction. Severall well-defined syndromes due to CMA have been identified, but in our experience these make up less than 5% of all children who suffer from hypersensitivity to milk proteins. These syndromes include the following:

- Milk-induced pulmonary disease [9]
- Allergic gastroenteropathy [10]
- Iron-losing enteropathy [11]
- Neonatal thrombocytopaenia - TAR [12]
- Neonatal thrombocytopaenia [13]
- Milk-induced colitis in infancy [14]

In recent studies employing a carefully standardized milk challenge procedure and conducted in a specialized hospital unit, we have documented a broad spectrum of symptoms and signs in children with CMA which have been elicited by milk ingestion [15] (Table 1). Entering this information into a computer data bank and subjecting it to cluster analysis, we were able to identify the following groups of patients with CMA.

Group 1: Patients develop acute perioral or generalized skin eruptions. One third of them have associated vomiting, wheezing and coughing or rhinitis following challenge, and some show acute stridor. Virtually all these patients have evidence of skin-sensitizing or circulating IgE antibodies to milk. Symptoms develop within 1 h of milk challenge.

Group 2: Patients show predominantly gastrointestinal reactions. A high incidence of acute vomiting and diarrhoea is recorded, and an unexpectedly high incidence of irritable or colicky behaviour is noted. Failure to thrive is commonly seen in this group. A low incidence of positive skin test and IgE antibodies to milk is found. IgA deficiency is common. Symptoms develop within 24 h of milk challenge.

Group 3: Patients have a high incidence of chronic skin eruptions, diarrhoea, respiratory problems and failure to thrive. Patients with skin problems show skin sensitivity to milk and high levels of IgE milk antibodies. Elevated levels of total IgM immunoglobulin are found in this population. Symptoms develop more than 24 h after milk challenge.

Colic or irritable behaviour, with or without other symptoms of CMA, was seen in nearly half of the 100 patients in this investigation, but

Table 1. Clinical features of 100 infants with proven CMA

Clinical feature[a]	Incidence
Gastrointestinal	
Vomiting	41
Diarrhoea	48
Colic	14
Colitis	4
Functional intestinal obstruction[b]	3
Generalized anaphylaxis[b]	
Stridor, collapse	2
Dermatological features	
Urticaria (general)	10
Angio-oedema	13
Circumoral lesions	26
Morbilliform eruptions	6
Eczema	13
Perianal eruptions	1
Respiratory	
Stridor (recurrent)	4
Rhinitis	21
Cough, wheeze	29
Tachypnoea	1
Nervous system	
Irritability[b]	40
Syncope (collapse alone)[b]	12
Convulsion[b]	2
Other manifestations	
Anemia[b]	2
Osteoporosis[b]	1
Severe failure to thrive[c]	22
Gross gastroesophageal reflux (radiological)[b]	6

[a] All symptoms elicited by challenge unless otherwise indicated.
[b] Features attributed to milk ingestion prior to formal challenge.
[c] Weight < 3rd percentile.

there were no significant differences in the incidence of this symptom among the three patient groups. However, there is evidence that one form of CMA does manifest itself in colic or irritable behaviour during infancy. JACOBSSON and LINDBERG [6], in a placebo-controlled study of colicky breast-fed infants, showed that half became asymptomatic when cow's milk was eliminated from the maternal diet, and that colic reappeared in two-thirds when the mothers were challenged with cow's milk protein. LOTHE et al. [7] showed that more than half of artificially fed colicky infants responded to elimination of cow's milk or soy milk from their diet. Evans et al. [8] were unable to confirm the value of avoiding cow's milk in breast-fed colicky infants; this study, however, can be criticized on the following grounds: (a) soy milk was used as a cow's milk substitute, and this can elicit colic symptoms in sensitized individuals; (b) the number of patients studied was small; (c) the duration of milk elimination from the maternal diet was too short to allow full evaluation of the role of milk protein avoidance in the treatment of colicky breast-fed infants. Further studies are required to define the frequency with which infants with colic symptoms respond to dietary manipulation.

Collectively these observations suggest that most children with CMA present in infancy and early childhood with one of the following clinical syndromes:

1. An anaphylactic response, e.g. urticaria, angio-oedema, acute stridor, wheeze or syncopal episode.
2. Episodic severe vomiting and/or diarrhoea.
3. Chronic ill health with multi-system disease associated with failure to thrive and/or chronic diarrhoea, eczema, bronchitic and wheezing symptoms.
4. Severe colic.

These clinical syndromes have been identified primarily in artificially fed infants, but there is increasing evidence from placebo-controlled double-blind studies that maternally ingested cow's milk and egg can be excreted in breast milk to elicit the anaphylactic, eczematous, and colic syndromes described above [16, 19, 20].

Uncommon Clinical Presentations of CMA

In clinical practice there are three less common situations in which the diagnosis of CMA may have to be considered:

1. The child with a positive skin test and elevated level of IgE antibodies to cow's milk.
2. The child with an anaphylactic reaction to egg or other food substance.
3. The child with chronic failure to thrive, diarrhoea, and essentially normal jejunal biopsy findings.

Positive Skin Test and Elevated Level of IgE Antibodies to Cow's Milk. A recently completed study of 120 infants and young children (median age, 24 months) with suspected CMA included a total of 135 milk challenges of which 68 were positive and 67 negative (unpublished data). Patients underwent a skin prick test (SPT) with a commercially available whole cow's milk extract, and the size of a weal diameter compared to histamine acid phosphate 1 mg/ml and graded from 0 to >4. A radioallergosorbent test (RAST) to cow's milk was carried out with commercially available reagents in the routine laboratory manner and graded according to manufacturer's directions.

SPT scores were dichotomized (partition between 0–2 vs 3, 4, >4) according to the level of reaction, as were the serum IgE antibodies to cow's milk as measured by RAST. Discriminant analysis showed both the SPT and the RAST scores to be statistically significant discriminators between milk-allergic and non-milk-allergic children ($p < 0.05$). However, when scores were dichtotomized with a partition point between 3 and 4, discriminant analysis showed that only the SPT discriminated milk-allergic from non-milk-allergic cases ($p < 0.005$). SPT specificity, i.e. the incidence of true negative results obtained when applied to children in whom CMA was not demonstrated, was 100%. On the other hand, SPT sensitivity, i.e. the incidence of true positive results when applied to patients known to be milk-challenge positive, was 47.1%. The overall efficiency of the test was 73%.

Based on the information generated in infants and young children in this study, the predictive value of a highly positive SPT (values of 4 or greater) is 100%. The predictive value of scores between 0 and 3 is 65%; this means that nearly four out of ten children with this level of skin test reactivity to milk in fact have CMA. In the clinical context, this means that the SPT can be a very useful diagnostic tool; most children with a SPT score of ⩾4 have a history of an anaphylactic or rapidly responding reaction to formal milk challenge. These make up about 25% of all children with CMA.

Table 2. Associated food intolerance in 100 children with CMA

Egg	40/77	Peanut	13/26
Orange	27/56	Chicken	7/75
Soy	32/75	Lamb	2/85
Chocolate	14/22	Beef	9/79
Wheat	12/88	Fish	6/69
Casein hydrolysate	11/54	Tomato	5/31

Anaphylactic Reaction to Egg or Other Food Substance. Occasionally CMA is diagnosed in an infant referred for evaluation of an acute anyphylactic reaction to an unrelated food, particularly egg, soy or peanut. This emphasizes the frequency with which allergic reactions to unrelated food antigens occur in children with CMA. Table 2 presents the frequency with which we have seen allergic reactions to other foods in children with CMA. Clinically, this means that if a hypersensitivity reaction to one food is identified, the possibility of hypersensitivity to other foods should also be considered.

It is of interest that children with anaphylactic IgE hypersensitivity to one food frequently show a non-IgE and non-immediate clinical response to unrelated dietary antigens. It remains to be investigated whether this is an effect of the different intensity of exposure to different dietary antigens during periods of immune vulnerability in infancy which influences the pattern of immune response that we have documented in CMA infants [21]. Furthermore, we have observed a few children whose clinical and immunological response to cow's milk altered over several years from that of an anaphylactic IgE hypersensitivity in infancy to that of non-IgE delayed type of onset in later childhood (personal observation). In our highly selected milk-allergic population it is worth observing that some patients appear to tolerate soy milk and casein hydrolysate preparations for several weeks or even months before they begin to develop clinical hypersensitivity reactions to them.

Chronic Failure to Thrive, Diarrhoea and Essentially Normal Jejunal Biopsy. Jejunal biopsy findings resembling coeliac disease and partial villous atrophy have been documented in patients with CMA [22], but this degree of change is relatively uncommon. More frequently, jejunal biopsies in children with CMA-induced diarrhoea and failure to thrive show minimal or no abnormality upon light microscopy. In a recent study [23] of 13 infants who were asymptomatic on a milk-free diet and experienced the onset of symptoms within 24 h after milk challenge, a range of changes in jejunal biopsy findings and lactase levels were observed. The biopsy changes were recorded by a histopathologist who did not know the diagnosis of individuals at the time of scoring the pathological lesions; structural changes were graded as showing normal appearance or mild, moderate, or severe change, as described by Townley et al. [24]. Table 3 gives the results. Three children showed significant changes on biopsy after milk challenge; more than half of those who showed an adverse clinical response to milk ingestion did not show any significant lesion on the post-challenge biopsy specimen.

Table 3. Effect of milk ingestion on jejunal histopathology in CMA

Clinical group	Patient	Challenge symptom	Histological abnormality[a]		Lactase in ≥1.1 unit/g wet weight	
			Before	After	Before	After
I	A	U, AE	Mild	Mild	2.4	2.6
I	B	AE	N	Mild	3.7	5.8
I	C	U, AE, V, D	N	N	1.9	2.9
I	D	Rash, D	Mild	Mild	1.5	2.0
I	E		N	N	3.2	2.4
II	F	D	Mild	Moderate	3.3	1.3
II	G	V, D	N	N	2.1	1.1
II	H	V, D	N	Severe	2.1	0.3
II	I	V, D	N	Moderate	3.6	1.6
III	J	D	N	N	4.3	4.7
III	K	V, D	N	N	4.5	5.0
III	L	D	N	N	3.2	4.5
III	M	Wh, C, D	N	N	1.0	0.5

U, Urticaria; AE, angio-oedema; V, vomiting; D, diarrhoea; Wh, wheezing.

[a] Mild, moderate, or severe according to TOWNLEY et al. [24]

Table 4. Clinical features of food allergy

Feature	Skin	Gastrointestinal	Mixed	Colic
Milk	++	++	++	+
Wheat	±	++	±	?
Egg	+++	+	++	+
Soy	+	++	++	+
Casein	+	+	+	+

Subsequently we have identified a number of children with chronic diarrhoea and essentially normal jejunal histopathology who responded to milk avoidance. Not infrequently these children showed non-IgE hypersensitivity intolerance to other common dietary antigens which needed to be excluded from their diet to induce remission of chronic diarrhoea.

CMA as a Model of Food Allergy

Our detailed studies have been confined to allergic reactions to cow's milk protein in infants and young children, but preliminary evidence which we have obtained suggests that a similar spectrum of clinical responses is seen in children with allergic reactions to other foods. Table 4 summarizes the patterns of clinical reactions that we have observed to some other common foods which we have attributed to allergic reactions (personal observation). It is worth highlighting several points in these findings. Anaphylactic reactions to egg is readily diagnosed, but the slow onset of vomiting and/or diarrhoea several hours after egg ingestion and the slower development of asthma or eczematous lesions over 12–24 h are less frequently recognized. The pathogenic role of wheat gluten in coeliac disease is well documented, but we have also identified a number of children with non-coeliac wheat allergy. These develop diarrhoea and abdominal pains within 12–72 h of commencing wheat ingestion and have normal jejunal biopsy findings when symptomatic (unpublished data). We have not defined the range of wheat antigens to which these patients are sensitized, but we have evidence to suggest that some children with IgE-associated wheat allergy respond to the non-gluten fractions of wheat, unlike children with coeliac disease [25]. The significance of these findings at this stage is unclear. With the increasing use of soy milk and casein hydrolysate preparations in infancy we are starting to identify a spectrum of clinical reactions in children allergic to these substances similar to that in the case of CMA.

Our studies concerning the diagnostic significance of skin tests have been confined to CMA, but in carefully conducted studies Bock et al. [26] and Sampson and Albergo [27] have described the value of skin tests to other foods. Histological lesions on jejunal biopsy may be elicited following the ingestion of soy milk and wheat in some children with allergy to these substances, but our preliminary findings suggest that the diagnosis of hypersensitivity reactions to milk and other foods should not rest entirely on the demonstration of such lesions. The diagnosis of allergy to these substances still rests on a reproducible clinical response to challenge conducted under controlled clinical conditions. Ideally, a placebo-controlled procedure should be undertaken, however the relatively large volumes of substances needed to elicit delayed-onset reactions precludes a satisfactory placebo challenge being devised. Small-bowel biopsy does have an important role in excluding other non-immune causes of gastrointestinal disease.

Concluding Remarks

A broad range of symptoms attributable to food allergy in infancy and childhood has been documented. In children with an anaphylactic type of reaction to foods, very high levels of skin test reactivity is diagnostic of a continuing hypersensitivity to the substances tested, but in all other cases diagnosis rests on a reproducible adverse response to food challenge. In cases in which symptoms such as failure to thrive and chronic diarrhoea are prominent, a jejunal biopsy is necessary to exclude non-immune causes of gastrointestinal disease. It is hoped that the development of other simple laboratory tests will facilitate diagnosis of the non-anaphylactic type of reaction to foods. Until such tests are available, the diagnosis of delayed-onset adverse reactions to foods should be regarded with some scepticism. With increasing awareness that dietary deprivation can represent one form of child abuse, the onus is on allergists to define more precisely the range of symptoms which they are prepared to attribute to food allergy.

Acknowledgments. The author gratefully acknowledges the assistance of Sisters ALISON DUKE and JENNY BROWN and the secretarial assistance of JOAN SEDMAK.

References

1. Pearson DJ, Rix KJ, Bentley ST (1983) Food allergy: how much in the mind? Lancet 1:1259
2. Warner JO, Hathaway MJ (1984) Allergic form of Meadow's syndrome. Arch Dis Child 59:151
3. Jacobsson I, Lindberg T (1979) A prospective study of cow's milk protein intolerance in Swedish infants. Acta Paediatr Scand 68:853
4. Gerrard JW, McKenzie J, Goluboff N, Garson J, Maningos C (1973) Cow's milk allergy: prevalence and manifestations in an unselected series of newborn. Acta Paediatr Scand [Suppl] 243:3
5. Roy C, Dubois R (1973) Gastroenterologic disorders. In: Steihm RE, Fulginiti VA (eds) Immunologic disorders in infants and children. Saunders, Philadelphia
6. Matthew TS, Soothill JF (1970) Complement activation after milk feeding in children with cow's milk allergy. Lancet ii:893
7. Parish WE (1971) Detection of reaginic and short-term sensitizing anaphylactic or anaphylactoid antibodies to milk in sera of allergic and normal persons. Clin Allergy 1:369
8. Borrone C, Dagna-Bricarelli F, Massimo L, Fossati-Gugliemoni A, Durand F (1970) Lymphocyte transformation in milk allergy. Acta Paediatr Scand 59:449

9. Heiner DC, Sears JW (1960) Chronic respiratory diseases associated with multiple circulating precipitins to cow's milk. Am J Dis Child 100:500
10. Waldemann TA, Wochner RD, Laster L et al. (1967) Allergic gastroenteropathy: a cause of excessive gastrointestinal protein loss. N Engl J Med 276:761
11. Wilson JF, Heiner DC, Lahey ME (1964) Milk induced gastrointestinal bleeding in infants with hypocromic and microcytic anaemia. JAMA 189:122
12. Whitfield MF, Barr DG (1976) Cow's milk allergy in the syndrome of thrombocytopaenia with absent radius. Arch Dis Child 51:337
13. Jones RH (1977) Congenital thrombocytopaenia and milk allergy. Arch Dis Child 52:744
14. Gryboski JD, Burkle F, Hillman R (1966) Milk induced colitis in the infant. Pediatrics 38:299
15. Hill DJ, Ford RPK, Shelton MJ, Hosking CS (1984) A study of 100 infants and young children with cow's milk allergy. Clin Rev Allergy 2:125
16. Jakobsson I, Lindberg T (1983) Cow's milk proteins cause infantile colic in breast fed infants: a double-blind crossover study. Pediatrics 71 (2):268
17. Lothe L, Lindberg T, Jakobsson I (1982) Cow's milk formula as a cause of infantile colic: a double-blind study. Pediatrics 70 (1):7.
18. Evans RW, Fergusson DM, Allardyce RA, Taylor B (1981) Maternal diet in infantile colic in breast fed infants. Lancet 1:1340
19. Warner JD (1980) Food allergy in fully breast fed infants. Clin Allergy 10:133
20. Cant AJ, Bailes JA, Marsden RA (1986) Effect of maternal dietary exclusions on breast fed infants with eczema: two controlled studies. Br Med J 293:231
21. Firer MA, Hosking CS, Hill DJ (1981) Effect of antigen load on development of milk antibodies in infants allergic to milk. Br Med J 283:693
22. Manuel PD, Walker-Smith JA, France NE (1979) Patchy enteropathy. Gut 20:211
23. Hill DJ, Davidson GP, Cameron DJ, Barnes GL (1979) The spectrum of cow's milk allergy in childhood. Acta Paediatr Scand 68:847
24. Townley RRW, Khaw KT, Schwachman H (1965) Quantitative assay of disaccharidase activities of small intestinal mucosal biopsy specimens in infancy and childhood. Pediatrics 36:911
25. Hill DJ, Baldo BA, Wrigley CW (1982) Immunoglobulin E antibodies to ingested cereal flour components: studies with sera from subjects with asthma and eczema. Clin Allergy 12:63
26. Bock SA et al. (1978) Appraisal of skin tests with food extracts for the diagnosis of food hypersensitivity. Clin Allergy 8:559
27. Sampson HA, Albergo R (1984) Comparison of results of skin tests, RAST, and double-blind, placebo-controlled food challenges in children with atopic dermatitis. J Allergy Clin Immunol 74:26

Gastrointestinal Manifestations of Food Allergy in Childhood

H. K. Harms and R. M. Bertele-Harms

Reliable data on the frequency of food allergy and its gastrointestinal manifestations in childhood can only be gained by comprehensive, prospective field studies. Furthermore, the definition of allergic reactions to food depends very much on the experience and opinion of the individual clinician, and this considerably influences the reported incidence and type of symptoms. Since no study on this subject has been conducted in the Federal Republic of Germany, we must rely on studies in neighbouring countries, such as those of JACOBSSON and LINDBERG in Malmö [1]. In a careful prospective study based on the results of well-defined elimination/challenge procedures, they reported a frequency of 1.9% in the 1st year of life. The most frequent combinations of symptoms were gastrointestinal and skin. Two-thirds of symptomatic infants showed gastrointestinal symptoms, such as colic, vomiting and diarrhoea. The main antigen was cow's milk protein, followed by soya, egg, fish, organges, tomatoes and cereals. Among the 20 allergic patients only two showed failure to thrive, indicating malabsorption following damage to the small-intestinal mucosa.

If the figures from Malmö are accepted as a basis, then the prevalence of food allergy with gastrointestinal symptoms is 10 times more frequent than coeliac disease and 20 times than cystic fibrosis.

In contrast to the Malmö study, patients in our clinic during the 1970s with protracted diarrhoea and severe failure to thrive predominated. This was a highly selected group of patients and characteristic of the majority of gastroenterologic clinics in Europe at that time. The patients were, almost without exception, exposed to a variety of cow's milk formulas, to which they reacted with diarrhoea and vomiting, generally within 1 h. The majority had lost substantial weight on admission and were considered as patients with intractable diarrhoea.

In our opinion, we are considering a single disease entity which, if neither recognized nor fully evaluated, will become grave and will involve long hospitalization of several weeks to months and sometimes even years. Thus, it is first necessary to consider this patient group in detail.

Particularly striking in their diet history was that hardly any of the children had been breast fed for longer than 1 week. A large majority received cow's milk formulas from birth; 60% became ill in the first 2 weeks of life, 23% in the following 2 weeks (Figs. 1, 2). The most fre-

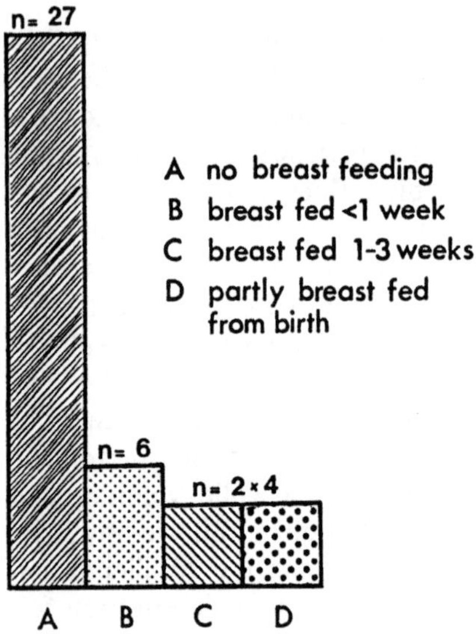

Fig. 1. Dietary history in 41 infants with cow's milk allergy and severe protracted diarrhoea

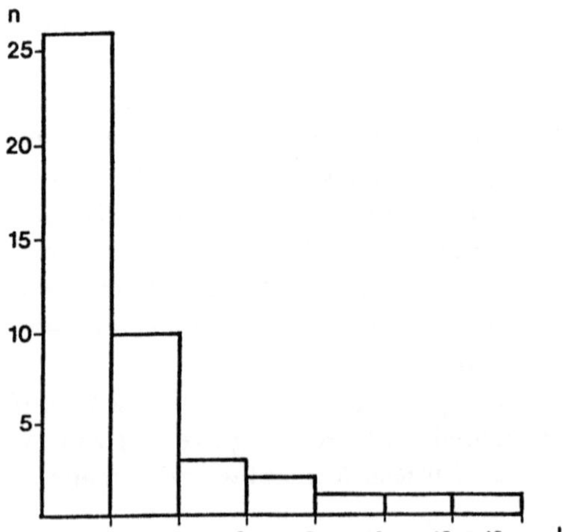

Fig. 2. Age at first symptoms in 44 infants with cow's milk allergy and severe protracted diarrhoea

quent symptom was diarrhoea, of various degrees (Table 1). Stools were loose to watery and often contained mucous. Macroscopically bloody diarrhoea was observed in only one patient. Vomiting was the second most frequent symptom, followed by anorexia and infections of the upper respiratory tract. Skin symptoms were relatively seldom. Occult blood was observed in all patients whose stools were analysed (Table 2). The frequently high platelet count of up to 800000/mm^3 stood out among the remaining results of laboratory investigations. A pathogen, predominantly of the *Escherichia coli* group, was found once in the stools of one-third of the infants; the significance of this remains uncertain. At that time, stools were not routinely investigated for rotavirus infection.

The basis for the prevailing scepticism in the 1970s concerning the diagnosis of cow's milk allergy or intolerance is clearly presented in Fig. 3, which shows a typical course with frequently unsuccessful di-

Table 1. Symptoms of infants with cow's milk allergy and severe protracted diarrhoea

Diarrhoea	45/46	98%
Watery mucous	41/45	
Visible blood	1/45	
Purulent	1/45	
Vomiting	33/46	72%
Dehydration	23/46	50%
Annorexia	10/46	22%
Fever	8/46	17%
Upper respiratory infections	11/46	24%
Dermatitis	8/46	17%
Abdominal distension	25/46	59%
Pallor	10/46	22%

Table 2. Laboratory results on infants with cow's milk allergy and severe protracted diarrhoea

Microcytic anaemia (haemoglobin <10 g/dl)	6/46	13%
Bands (>10%)	12/46	26%
Eosinophilic granulocytes (>500/mm)	8/46	17%
Platelets (>350000/mm)	18/46	39%
Total proteins (<5.5 g/dl)	8/46	17%
Occult blood in stools	8/8	100%
Pathogenic stool cultures	12/33	36%
(11× enteropathogenic *Escherichia coli*, 1× salmonellosis)		

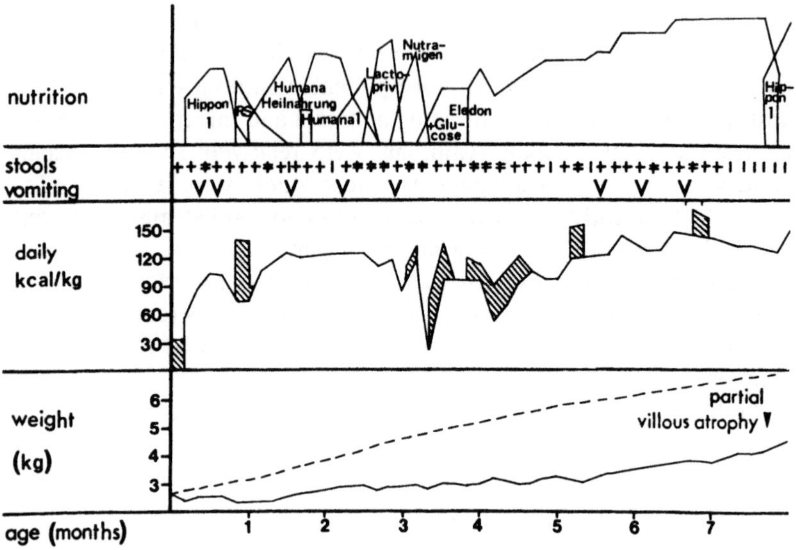

Fig. 3. Example of dietary mistreatment in a young infant with cow's milk allergy and severe protracted diarrhoea. *Hippon, Humana, Eledon:* cow's milk formulas; *Lactopriv:* soya-based formula; *RS:* rice-based formula. *V*, Vomiting; ⧺, diarrhoea; |, normal stods; *shadings*, parenteral nutrition; *dashed line*, third percentile

etary trials. The young infant was admitted still in a good condition shortly after birth and then received various cow's and soya milk formulas, as well as a casein hydrolysate. These challenges triggered more frequent and prolonged episodes of diarrhoea and increased malnutrition. Highly wasted infants then become the rule (Fig. 4). Nearly 50% of infants were treated with cow's milk formulas for longer than 2 months following the onset of symptoms, and one-fourth for longer than 3 months (Fig. 5). The average period before cow's milk was withdrawn from their diet was 10.4 weeks. This "mistreatment" produced an iatrogenic weight loss of up to 7 standard deviations below the mean (Fig. 6). All the biopsied patients in Fig. 6 showed more or less marked injury of the small intestinal mucosa. Among these, partial villous atrophy, i.e. the "patchy" lesion (Fig. 7), was represented as frequent as a subtotal villous atrophy, which was indistinguishable from the mucosa in untreated coeliac disease. The infants, who received a cow's milk containing diet for more than 8 weeks were, on average, more markedly wasted and required longer hospitalization than those with a shorter history. Furthermore, two-thirds of those severely ill demonstrated a flat mucosa in comparison to only one-third among the remainder

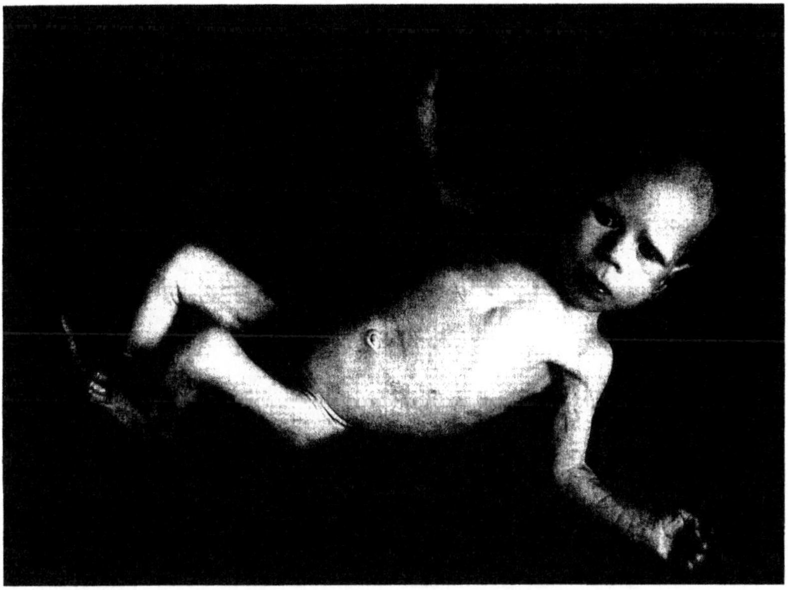

Fig. 4. Example of a 4-month-old, highly wasted and mistreated infant

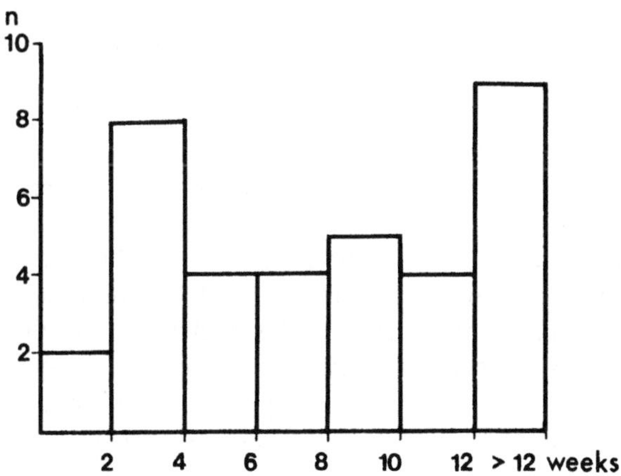

Fig. 5. Interval between first symptoms and cow's milk free diet in 36 infants

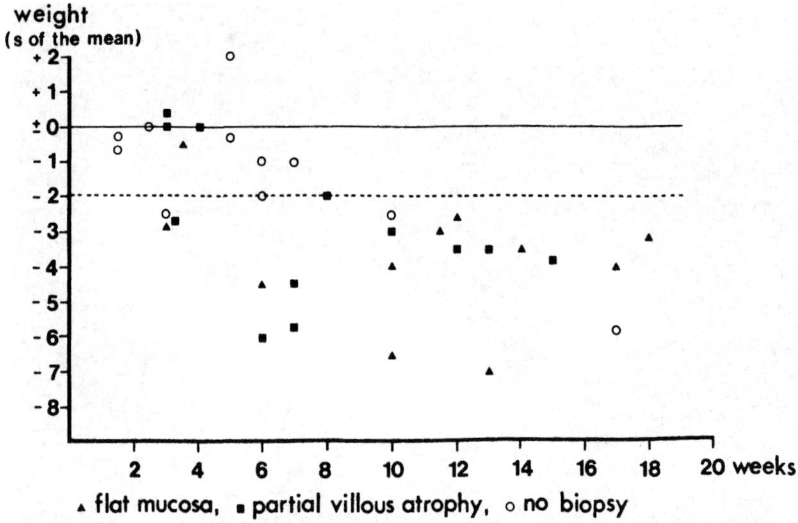

Fig. 6. Standard deviation of weight in 34 infants on continued cow's milk feeding *after* onset of symptoms. *Dotted line*, third percentile

(Fig. 6). Although not conclusive, this may indicate that the long-lasting catabolic situation had, in addition, an aggravating effect on the severity of the mucosal injury. The mucosa in these infants is thinner than in coeliac patients [2].

The clinical picture and course of the illness, together with the changes in the small-intestinal mucosa, indicate an ominous vicious circle which would be further exacerbated by the noxious cow's milk protein and can lead to a secondary bacterial contamination of the small intestine (Fig. 8). It need hardly be stated that the mucosa in the catabolic situation cannot repair itself. A non-intact epithelial layer and mucosal barrier does not offer sufficient protection against the various dietary antigens, bacteria and viruses. This may be aggravated by the reduced capacity of a damaged intestinal epithelium to secrete sufficient secretory elements to form sIgA and sIgM, which are of particular importance in the local immunological defense system.

What evidence can be found that cow's milk proteins damage the small intestinal mucosa, and what observations indicate that immunological processes are involved?

Various investigators have been able to demonstrate that the small-intestinal mucosa recovers during a cow's milk free diet and is damaged again when reexposed to small amounts of cow's milk [3, 4]. The re-

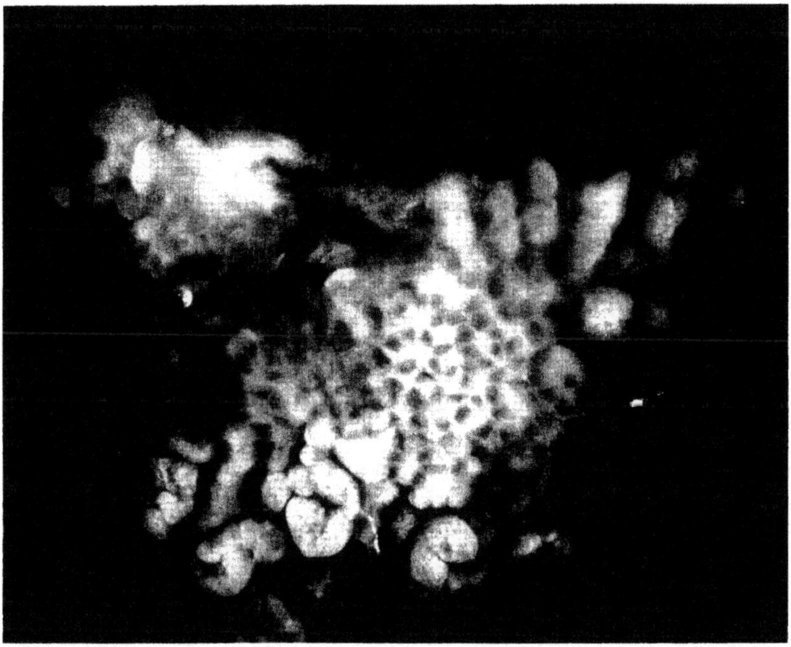

Fig. 7. "Patchy" lesion of the biopsied small-intestinal mucosa with combination of totally flat areas and partially "atrophic" stunted villi. ($\times$25)

newed villous injury could be shown both morphologically and functionally, for example, in deterioration in the 1-h D-xylose test [5, 6]. The most probable explanation of these mucosal reactions is as an immunological process. Although even healthy, non-breast-fed infants show antibodies in serum against cow's milk proteins during their 1st year, these are nonetheless markedly higher in infants with cow's milk protein allergy and damaged mucosa [7, 8]. Accordingly, evidence of particularly high antibody titres against cow's milk proteins is of certain diagnostic value. However, high antibody titres to cow's milk proteins do not permit any conclusion as to the aetiology of the involvement of antibodies in the pathogenesis of mucosal damage, for such high antibody titres have also been found in untreated coeliac disease [7]. More evidence for an immunological genesis of mucosal injury comes from (a) the observation of an increase in the number of IgA- and IgM-containing plasma cells [9, 10] and specific antibodies [11] in the lamina propria following a challenge by cow's milk proteins and (b) the demonstration of immune complex deposits on the basal membrane [12], which corresponds

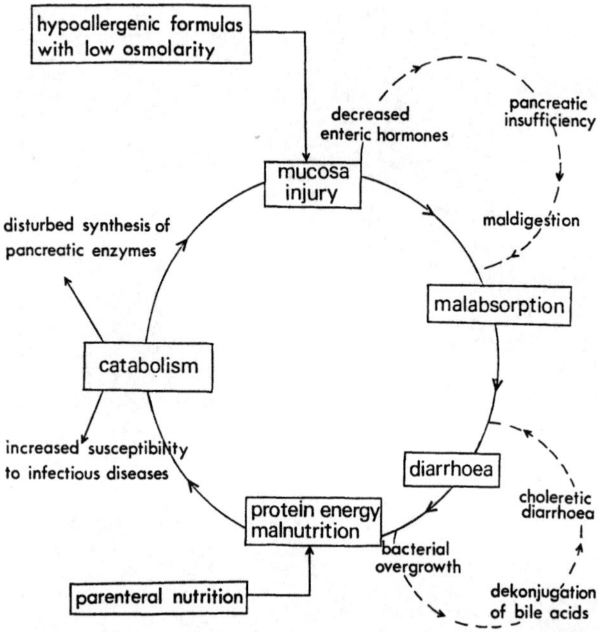

Fig. 8. Ominous vicious circle in mistreated infants with cow's milk allergy and severe protracted diarrhoea and the therapeutic possibilities for its interruption

to an Arthus-type III inflammatory reaction. Following milk challenge a higher amount of specific cow's milk protein antibodies are excreted into the intestinal lumen [13, 14]. Furthermore, high IgE antibodies to cow's milk proteins, which have been demonstrated in the serum of patients [7], could additionally induce an early reaction to a cow's milk challenge. Finally, an increase of intra-epithelial lymphocytes following challenge [15, 16] may offer further evidence for the provocation of immunological reactions to cow's milk proteins.

All the observed immunological reactions to cow's milk protein challenges support the conclusion that these proteins are immunologically involved in inducing and maintaining small-intestinal mucosal injury. This does not mean that cow's milk proteins are the primary cause, as bacterial or viral infections, e.g. the rotavirus infection, can equally well cause the primary mucosal damage which is followed by the immunological reaction against the foreign proteins [4, 17]. The immunological incompetence of the newborn and the lack of protection from the breast milk certainly favours the adherence of bacteria to the intestinal wall

[18]. In most cases, the pathogen responsible for the mucosal damage cannot be identified, for the search is begun too late, if at all.

As soya protein formulas are frequently used as a substitute in cow's milk allergy, it is not surprising that soya proteins have become other major allergens in infantile food allergy which may cause identical small intestinal mucosal lesions [19, 20]. The example in Fig. 9 shows the protraction of mucosal damage, originally induced by cow's milk proteins, by giving soya milk. It may be stated, retrospectively, that we did not then recognize soya protein intolerance as such but, at the same time, had hardly any alternative nourishment at our disposal.

The ominous vicious circle accompanied by severe wasting in the infant can be interrupted in only two ways (Fig. 8). The first, and most important, is to bring the organism out of a catabolic and into an anabolic situation. This can scarcely be obtained with oral feeding alone, considering the serious damage to the mucosa and its insufficient absorptive capacity. Very seriously ill infants therefore require, first of all, a parenteral nutrition through a central venous catheter; this is accompanied by considerable risks, such as catheter sepsis or thrombosis of the major vessels. Nevertheless, it is important to start oral feeding from the very beginning with a small amount of a suitable diet, i.e. one which does not release immunological reactions, is easily absorbed and is hypo-osmotic. Recovery is apparently accelerated by the very contact of food on the damaged small intestinal epithelium [21–23].

Freshly collected or temporally deep-frozen breast milk proved most effective (Table 3) [24, 25]. Interestingly, the secondary lactase deficiency apparently played no important role. The theoretical disadvantage is outweighed by the outstanding properties of breast milk. These consist not only in its immunological qualities but also in its excellent nutritional quality. It possesses, itself, a high lipolytic activity and has a low osmolarity, and its constituents, e.g. fat, iron, zinc and calcium, are particularly well absorbed. Our Finish colleagues reported similar success with fresh breast milk [26].

Table 3. The 84 dietary regimens in 41 patients with severe protracted diarrhoea

Diet	Successes	Failures	Success rate
Soya formula	13	17	43%
Casein hydrolysate	16	15	52%
Meat-based formula	5	4	55%
Human milk	12	2	85%

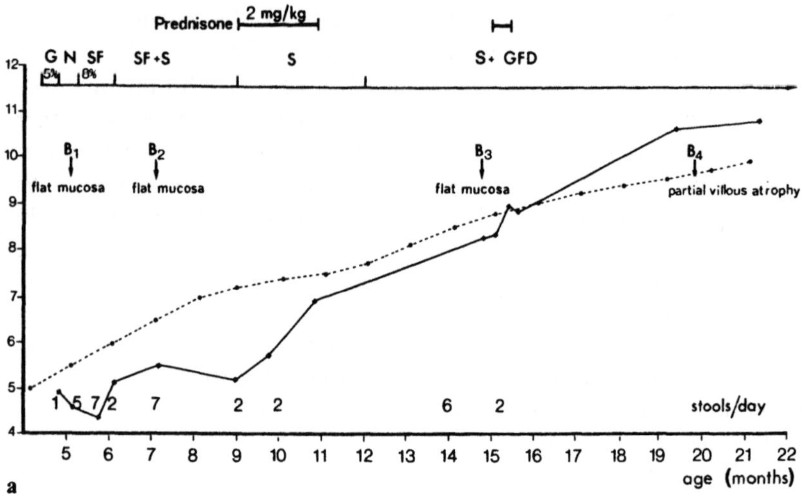

a

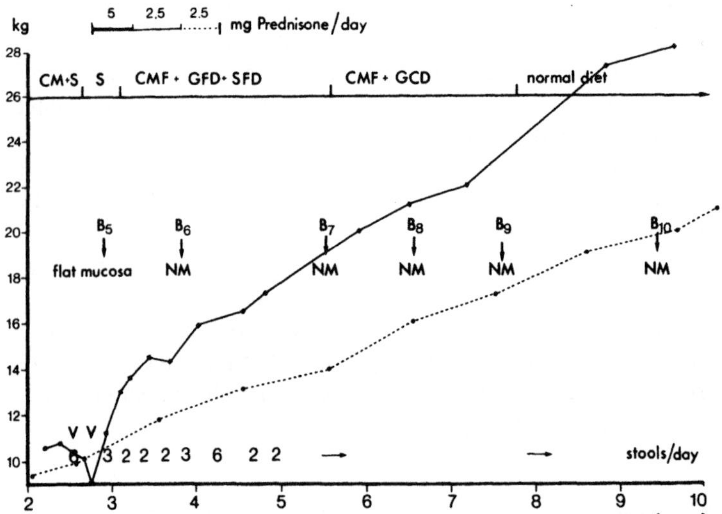

b

Fig. 9 a, b. Clinical and small-intestinal course in a child with severe protracted diarrhoea caused by cow's milk proteins and soya proteins. **a** Early. **b** Later. *G*, Glucose; *N*, Nutramigen; *S*, soya formula; *SF*, stepwise feeding (glucose 8%, casein hydrolysate, fat); *GFD*, gluten-free diet; *CM*, cow's milk; *SFD*, soya-free diet; *GCD*, gluten-containing diet; *B*, biopsy; *NM*, normal mucosa; *V*, vomiting; *dotted line*, third percentile

What Constitutes the Excellent Immunological Properties of Breast Milk? Although breast milk is rich in inflammation-suppressing properties, it is poor in initiators and mediators of inflammatory reactions [27]. The coagulation and the fibrinolytic systems as well as kallikrein are scarcely present in breast milk. The complement is much lower than in peripheral blood. Furthermore, IgG, the main activator of the complement system, is also low. In addition, no IgE is present in human milk.

The pronounced, important role of secretory IgA in breast milk, which gains its particular significance over the enteromammalian circulation, is not disputed. It prevents micro-organisms from binding to the surface of the intestinal mucosa, neutralizes their toxins and the virulence factors of micro-organisms and suppresses the chemotaxis of neutrophils. In addition, specific IgA antibodies reduce antigen absorption through the intestinal wall. Lactoferrin binds iron from bacteria and suppresses the complement system. Lysozyme limits the chemotaxis of neutrophilic granulocytes and the formation of oxygen radicals in leucocytes. α-1-antichymotrypsin and α-1-antitrypsin neutralize such inflammatory enzymes as leucocyte proteinases. α-2-Glycoprotein suppresses the formation of lymphocytes. Arylsulphatase degrades leucotrienes and histaminase histamine. α-Tocopherol, cystein and ascorbic acid are scavangers of oxygen radicals, and the catalase destroys hydrogen superoxide. All these properties have been demonstrated in human milk.

The cytotoxic abilities of breast milk are minimal. In addition, human milk contains neither thrombocytes nor effector leucocytes such as basophiles, mastocytes or eosinophilic granulocytes. Also, the oligosaccharides in breast milk protect against infection insofar as they act almost as receptor analogues for certain bacteria-binding structures on the epithelial cells. This has been demonstrated for pneumococci and epithelial cells of the respiratory tract. Finally, breast milk contains an epithelial growth factor which positively influences the growth of the mucosa. This strengthens the mucosal barrier against infection.

The observation that fresh human milk is the best therapeutic substance for severe cow's milk allergy, with damage to the small-intestinal mucosa, completes our understanding of this illness. It is a *breast milk deficiency disease* in which cow's milk proteins coincidentally produce or maintain damage to the mucosa. Instead of cow's milk proteins, the damage-producing proteins could be soya, as shown above, as well as fish or egg [28]. The illness can be prevented by exclusive breast feeding for at least 3 months.

As noted above, no infant with such a breast milk deficiency was identified in the prospective Malmö study on the frequency of cow's milk allergy. Even then, in 1981, more than 45% of mothers there fully breast fed their infants for at least 3 months. At the same time, in Munich only 5% of mothers breast fed for 3 months or longer. The later investigation was repeated in 1986 (I. BAUMANN, Local Health Service, Munich). In the meantime, the frequency of breast feeding in Munich had come to match that in Malmö, with some 40% of mothers exclusively breast feeding their babies at 3 months (Fig. 10). As a consequence, we have been confronted with far fewer cases of severe cow's milk protein allergy with small-intestinal mucosal damage in the past few years.

As the incidence of this syndrome of servere cow's milk allergy with small-intestinal injury has markedly decreased, our attention has turned increasingly in recent years to the IgE-mediated allergies, in particular in infants exclusively breast fed.

The example presented in Fig. 11 shows a thriving infant who, at age 2 weeks, passed increasingly bloody, mucoid stools and suffered consequent anaemia. The results of bacteriological and virological investigations were negative. The bloody diarrhoea stopped only after the mother eliminated cow's milk proteins from her own diet. Endoscopy of the colon showed considerably inflamed mucosa and a small ulcer. Histologically, the inflamed mucosa contained an infiltrate with plasma cells.

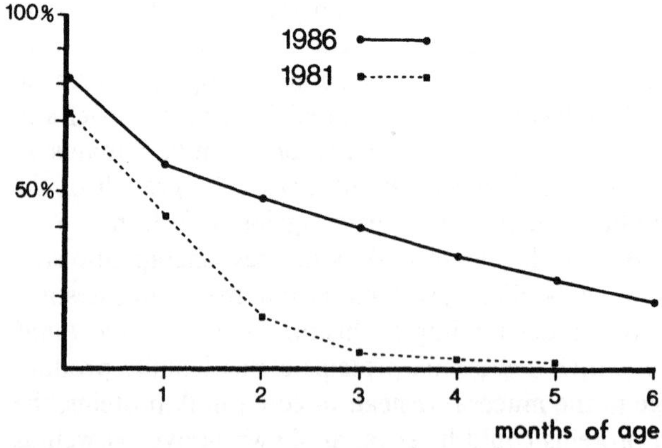

Fig. 10. Frequency of exclusive breast feeding in 1981 and 1986 in Munich. (Results obtained by I. Baumann)

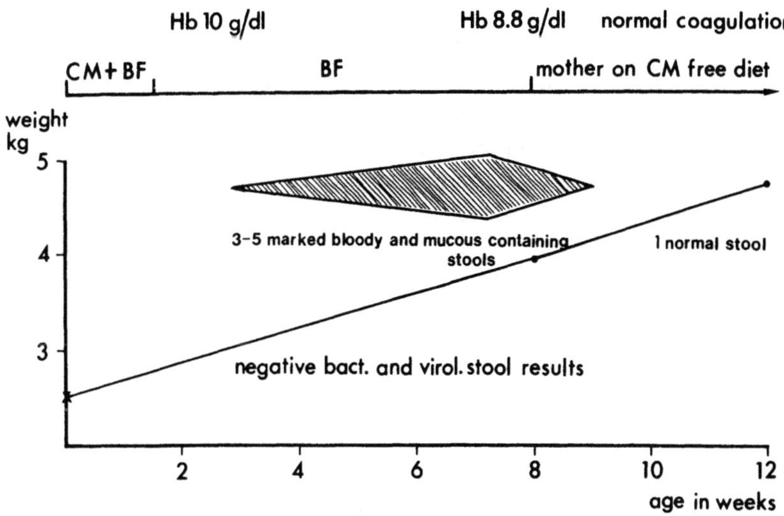

Fig. 11. Clinical course of an exclusively breast-fed infant with severe cow's milk protein induced colitis. *CM*, Cow's milk; *BF*, breast fed

Infantile colitis, caused by an allergy to the diet, is agreed to be the most frequent cause of non-infectious colitis in infancy and usually has its onset before the 4th month [29, 30]. Characteristic are soft, slimy, bloody stools and a good physical development. Histological findings are an infiltrate with plasma cells and eosinophilic granulocytes. Of published cases [31], 50% were exclusively breast fed. Challenges with the suspected protein in order to confirm the diagnosis are discouraged since massive bleeding and shock have been observed.

One of the most frequent gastrointestinal manifestations of an IgE-mediated food allergy is infantile colic, which is of particular practical significance. Jakobssen and her colleagues conducted important investigations on this topic [32, 33] and established that half the cases of colic, approximately 12% of infants, were released by cow's milk or soya proteins. At least one-third of these cases occur, on the other hand, during breast feeding and are released by traces of cow's milk protein as well as other proteins such as soya, egg and fish in the breast milk. The majority of these children come from atopic families.

The following example illustrates multiple allergic reactions to different antigens in breast milk. A male infant, aged 6.5 months, was brought to us having previously been exclusively breast fed. A severe atopic dermatitis, a most severe colic and mucoid diarrhoea developed from the 3rd month. On admission, he presented a sad picture, with itchy skin changes over the whole body, which in part bled and in part wept. His weight was below the third percentile. There was an oedema of the legs. Markedly abnormal were the laboratory findings: 21600 leucocytes with 27% eosinopohilic granulocytes, total protein of 3.4 g/dl, IgE of 2735 kU/l, and a radioallergosorbent test (RAST) for cow's milk, egg and fish being three- or four-fold positive. Interestingly, the cow's milk IgG antibody titres were also increased. Furthermore, the mother informed us that every time that she ate fish, the child reacted with explosive diarrhoea at the subsequent occassion of breast feeding. Exceptionally in this case, there was no atopic family history.

Another infant was similarly noteworthy. Likewise exclusively breast fed for 3 months, it showed a severe atopic dermatitis from the 1st month of age. The dermatitis deteriorated with cow's milk, soya and cereal formulas and other dietetic trials. A marked weeping and itchy, generalized eczema, as well as slimy stools and eyelid oedema, were observed on admission. Laboratory results were similar to those of the previous patient and showed 24% eosinophilic granulocytes, a reduction in total proteins to 29 g/l, a very high IgE (>800 kU/l), and four-fold positive RAST tests for cow's milk, egg and rye proteins. Interestingly, the geometric mean of IgG cow's milk antibodies and the titre for IgG gliadin antibodies were markedly increased. A biopsy of the small intestine revealed a morphologically normal mucosa with normal disaccharidase activities.

Disregarding for the moment the many unmistakable and easily treatable IgE-mediated food allergies with gastrointestinal involvement, we have recently been somewhat disturbed at the frequency with which we find pronounced IgE-mediated allergic reactions among exclusively breast-fed infants. Naturally, this will certainly not force us to doubt the value and significance of exclusive breast feeding during the first months of life. Nevertheless, it does accord with our low expectations concerning prevention of IgE-mediated reactions in young infants.

References

1. Jakobsson J, Lindberg T (1979) A prospective study of cow's milk protein intolerance in Swedish infants. Acta Paediatr Scand 68:853–859
2. Maluenda C, Phillips AD, Briddon A, Walker-Smith JA (1984) Quantitative analysis of small intestinal mucosa in cow's milk sensitive enteropathy. J Ped Gastr Nutr 3:349–356
3. Iyngkaran N, Robinson M, Prathap K et al. (1978) Cow's milk protein-sensitive

enteropathy. Combined clinical and histological criteria for diagnosis. Arch Dis Child 53:20-26
4. Walker-Smith J (1982) Cow's milk intolerance as a cause of postenteritis diarrhoea. J Pediatr Gastroenterol Nutr 1:163-173
5. Morin CL, Weber A, Buts JP et al. (1979) One-hour blood-xylose test in diagnosis of cow's milk protein intolerance. Lancet I:1102-1104
6. Iyngkaran N, Abidin Z (1982) One-hour blood xylose in the diagnosis of cow's milk protein sensitive enteropathy. Arch Dis Child 57:40-43
7. Bürgin-Wolff A, Signer E, Friess HM et al. (1980) The diagnostic significance of antibodies in various cow's milk proteins (fluorescent immunosorbent test). Eur J Pediatr 133:17-24
8. Stern M, Stupp W, Grüttner R (1982) Cow's milk protein antibodies determined by immunofluorescence (RIFT) in cow's milk protein intolerance and in controls. Monatsschr Kinderheilkd 130:556-561
9. Savilahti E (1973) Immunochemical study of the malabsorption syndrome with cow's milk intolerance. Gut 14:491-501
10. Pearson JR, Kingston D, Shiner M (1983) Antibody production to milk protein in the jejunal mucosa of children with cow's milk protein intolerance. Pediatr Res 17:406-412
11. Stern M, Dietrich R, Mueller J (1982) Small intestinal mucosa ion coeliac disease and cow's milk protein intolerance: morphometric and immunofluorescent studies. Eur J Pediatr 139:101-105
12. Shiner M (1981) Ultrastructural features of allergic manifestations in the small intestine of children. Scand J Gastroenterol (Suppl), 70:49-64
13. Savilahti E, Kuitunen P, Visakorpi JK (1981) Cow's milk allergy. In: Lebenthal E (ed) Textbook of gastroenterology and nutrition in infancy, vol 2. New York, Ravens, New York, pp 689-708
14. Shah PG, Freier S, Park BH et al. (1982) Pancreozymin and secretin enhance duodenal fluid antibody levels to cow's milk proteins. Gastroenterology 83:916-921
15. Kosnai I, Kuitunen P, Savilahti E et al. (1980) Cell kinetics in the jejunal crypt epithelium in malabsorption syndrome with cow's milk protein intolerance and in coeliac disease. Gut 21:1041-1046
16. Phillips AD, Rice SJ, France NE et al. (1979) Small intestine intraepithelial lympohocyte levels in cow's milk protein intolerance. Gut 20:509-512
17. Harrison M, Kilby A, Walker-Smith JA et al. (1976) Cow's milk protein intolerance: a possible association with gastroenteritis, lactose intolerance, and IgA deficiency. Br Med J I:1501-1504
18. Porter P (1979) Adoptive immunization by the neonate by breast factors. In: Ogra PL, Dayton D (eds) Immunology of breast milk. Ravens, New York, pp 197-206
19. Ament ME, Rubin CE (1972) Soy-protein - another cause of the flat intestinal lesion. Gastroenterology 62:227-234
20. Perkkio M, Savilahti E, Kuitunen P (1981) Morphometric and immunohistochemical study of jejunal biopsies from children with intestinal soy allergy. Eur J Pediatr 137:63-69
21. Greene HL, McCabe DR, Merenstein G (1975) Protacted diarrhea and malnutrition in infancy: changes in intestinal morphology and disaccharidase activities during treatment with total intravenous nutrition or oral elemental diets. J Pediatr 87:695-704

22. Weizman Z, Schmueli A, Deckelbaum RJ (1983) Continuous nasogastric drip elemental feeding. Am J Dis Child 137:253–255
23. Anonymus (1987) Chronic diarrhoea in children - a nutritional disease (Editorial). Lancet I:143–144
24. Harms HK, Bertele RM (1983) Die schwere protrahierte Säuglingsdiarrhoe ("intractable diarrhoea"). Monatsschr Kinderheilkd 131:428–435
25. MacFarlane PJ, Miller V (1984) Human milk in the management of protracted diarrhoea of infancy. Arch Dis Child 59:260–265
26. Kuitunen P, Visakorpi HK, Savilahti E, Pelkonen P (1975) Malabsorption syndrome with cow's milk intolerance. Arch Dis Child 50:351–356
27. Goldman AS, Thorpe LW, Goldblum RM, Hanson LA (1986) Anti-inflammatory properties of human milk. Acta Paediatr Scand 75:689–695
28. Vitoria JC, Camarero C, Sojo A et al. (1986) Enteropathy related to fish, rice, and chicken. Arch Dis Child 57:44–48
29. Lake AM, Whitington PF, Hamilton SR (1982) Dietary protein-induced colitis in breast-fed infants. J Pediatr 101:906–910
30. Jenkins HR, Pincott JR, Soothill HF et al. (1984) Food allergy: the major cause of infantile colitis. Arch Dis Child 59:326–329
31. Shorter RG (1987) Idiopathic inflammatory bowel disease: a form of food allergy? In: Brostoff J, Challcombe SJ (eds) Food allergy and intolerance. Bailliere, Tindall, London, pp 549–554
32. Jakobsson J, Lindberg T (1978) Cow's milk as a cause of infantile colic in breast-fed infants. Lancet 2:437–439
33. Jakobsson J, Lindberg T (1983) Cow's milk proteins cause infantile colic in breast-fed infants: a double-blind cross over study. Pediatrics 71:268–271

The Significance of Food Allergy in Atopic Dermatitis*

H. A. Sampson

Atopic dermatitis is an inflammatory skin disorder which frequently begins in early infancy. It is characterized by extreme pruritus, chronically relapsing course, and specific distribution. The rash is generally an erythematous, papulovesicular eruption, frequently with serous discharge and crusting, and progresses to a scaly, lichenified rash over time [1]. The distribution of the rash typically varies with age [2], involving the cheeks and extensor surfaces of the arms and legs in infancy, the flexor surfaces in the young child, and flexor surfaces, hands and feet in the teenage patient and young adult. Unlike most dermatoses, atopic dermatitis has no primary skin lesion but is identified by a constellation of symptoms. The classification system recently proposed by HANIFIN and RAJKA [3] has been generally accepted and provides suitable diagnostic criteria for the disorder.

BESNIER, a French physician, put forth the first comprehensive description of atopic dermatitis nearly a century ago [4]. He emphasized the hereditary nature of this disorder, its chronically recurring course, and its association with hayfever and asthma. He initially named the disorder *prurigo diathesique*, but it later became known as *Besnier prurigo*. WISE and SULZBERGER [5] further emphasized the relationship between atopic eczema, asthma, and hayfever by coining the term atopic dermatitis, the term generally used today. The incidence of atopic dermatitis has been increasing over the past 20 years and is now estimated to afflict between 2.4% and 8.3% of the pediatric population [6, 7].

The etiology of atopic dermatitis is unknown. Several physiological abnormalities have been noted [8]: (a) decreased itch threshold, (b) ab-

* Supported by grants AI24439 and AI00830 from the National Institute of Allergy and Infectious Diseases and by grants RR-30 and RR-00052 from the General Clinical Research Centers Program of the Division of Research Resources, National Institutes of Health. Data was managed and analyzed with CLINFO. The author is a recipient of the Allergic Diseases Academic Award, NIH.

normal cutaneous vascular responses, (c) increased transepidermal water loss, and (d) abnormal pharmacological responses, including β-adrenergic blockade. Abnormalities of both humoral and cellular immunity have been described in patients with atopic dermatitis and appear to vary with the severity of the clinical symptoms [9]: (a) elevated serum IgE, (b) defective delayed-type skin responsiveness to various antigens, (c) variably decreased lymphocyte response to mitogens, recall antigens, and alloantigens, (d) defective generation of cytotoxic T-lymphocyte response in vitro, and (e) variably decreased phagocytic capacity and chemotaxis of neutrophils and monocytes.

Although the association with allergy was noted by Besnier in his original description, the pathogenic role of allergy in this disorder has been debated for years. Circumstantial evidence suggest a significant role for an IgE-mediated mechanism(s) in atopic dermatitis: (a) two-thirds of patients have a positive family history of atopy [10], (b) 80%–90% of children have elevated serum IgE concentrations [11], (c) approximately 80% of children have positive immediate skin tests and radioallergosorbent tests (RAST) to various dietary and environmental allergens [2, 13], and (d) 50%–80% of children develop other atopic disorders, such as allergic rhinitis and asthma [14, 15]. However, the histologic findings of skin lesions have been considered inconsistent with an IgE-mediated mechanism(s). Skin biopsy specimens obtained from acute and chronic lesions of patients with atopic dermatitis reveal mononuclear round cell infiltrates, especially at the dermal-epidermal junction. Increased numbers of mast cells and Langerhans' cells (LC), and demyelination of superficial nerve endings were noted in chronic lesions. The presence of this monocytic and lymphocytic infiltrate has prompted many investigators to suggest a classic cell-mediated, type IV hypersensitivity reaction as the underlying cause of the eczematous skin lesion [16].

In the past 5 years, our studies have addressed the etiologic role of IgE-mediated food hypersensitivity in atopic dermatitis. Using double-blind placebo-controlled oral food challenges (DBPCFC), 183 patients with atopic dermatitis have been evaluated for food hypersensitivity. Subjects ranged in age from 3 months to 24 years, with a median age of 5.3 years. Family history was positive for atopic disease in 95% of subjects. Eighty-five patients (48%) also had allergic rhinitis and asthma, 51 (29%) had allergic rhinitis, 7 (4%) had asthma, and 40 (22%) had neither allergic rhinitis nor asthma. Serum total IgE concentration was elevated in 151 (85%) patients, with a median of 3400 IU/ml and a range of 1.5–45000 IU/ml (laboratory normal range, ±2 SD, was 5–621 IU/ml).

Patients enrolled in the study fulfilled the criteria of HANIFIN and RAJKA [3] for the diagnosis of atopic dermatitis. Prior to admitting subjects to the Clinical Research Center, patient history and previous allergy tests were reviewed. Foods administered in DBPCFC were selected on the basis of skin test (and RAST) results and/or a strongly suggestive history of food hypersensitivity. Foods selected for the challenge protocol were excluded from the patient's diet for 7–10 days prior to admission. In addition, oral corticosteroids were discontinued for at least 1 month and antihistamines for at least 1 week prior to admission.

Patients were tested to a battery of 20 food extracts (Greer Laboratories, Lenoir, North Carolina, USA) on the day of admission to standardize skin test data, confirm previous results, and determine which foods would be used in the DBPCFC. A venous line was established prior to initiating challenges for providing an open-line in case of a major anaphylactic reaction and for atraumatic serial blood sampling. DBPCFC were conducted as previously described [17]. Two challenges are performed each day, one containing the test food antigen and one containing placebo. The Clinical Research Unit dietician determined the order of all challenges, using a randomization scheme on the Unit's computer (CLINFO). Only the dietician was aware of the contents of the challenge. Over a 1-h period, up to 10 g dehydrated powdered food was administered in opaque capsules or in 100 ml juice. The initial dose was generally less than 500 mg and was increased in a step-wise fashion at 10- to 15-min intervals until the entire 10 g was consumed, or until a reaction occurred. Each challenge was evaluated and scored using a previously published symptom sheet [17]. Any patient experiencing a negative DBPCFC was fed the food openly prior to the time of discharge to ensure the accuracy of the blind challenge and to assure the patient (and parent) that the food could be consumed without difficulty. In over 700 food challenges performed to date, there have been four reactions during the open feeding following negative DBPCFC (<1% false-negative results). Three children, two aged 4 years and one aged 2 years, developed symptoms after drinking milk. One child developed cutaneous, nasal, and respiratory symptoms after consuming approximately 100 ml milk, one child developed cutaneous symptoms and periocular edema after ingesting about 80 ml, and the third child developed cutaneous, upper respiratory, and gastrointestinal symptoms after ingesting about 10 ml milk. The fourth child, aged 5 years, developed cutaneous, gastrointestinal, nasal, and respiratory symptoms after eating a standard portion of peas.

A total of 539 DBPCFC have been conducted in the initial evaluation of this group of children with atopic dermatitis. DBPCFC were not conducted in 31 instances because history revealed a "convincing" account of a major anaphylactic reaction. History was considered convincing when a patient experienced severe respiratory compromise (laryngeal edema and/or wheezing) and/or hypotension within minutes of ingesting an isolated food and required emergency care by a physician. In each case in which the challenge was not performed, the patient had a strongly positive prick skin test to the food in question: peanut, 17; egg, 5; fish, 4; milk, 2; soy, 1; beef, 1; and potato, 1. No patient experienced a severe anaphylactic reaction during DBPCFC, although several subjects required oral diphenhydramine for severe pruritus, and three patients required subcutaneous epinephrine for respiratory symptoms.

Of the 539 DBPCFC performed, 317 were interpreted as negative and 190 as positive. Cutaneous reactions developed in 164/190 instances (86%) and consisted of a pruritic, erythematous, macular or morbilliform rash. Symptoms confined exclusively to the skin occurred in only 36% of the reactions. Urticarial lesions were rarely seen and generally consisted of only two or three lesions. Intense pruritus resulted in scratching, which frequently led to superficial excoriations and occasionally to bleeding. Gastrointestinal symptoms were seen in 89/190 (47%) of the reactions even though a history of gastrointestinal symptoms was rarely elicited from the patients. The gastrointestinal symptoms that were seen consisted of nausea, abdominal pain, or both, plus vomiting, diarrhea, or both. Respiratory symptoms involving primarily the upper respiratory tract were seen in 38/190 (20%) of these with positive DBPCFC. Respiratory symptoms included nasal congestion, rhinorrhea, sneezing, stridor, and/or wheezing.

Except in one patient, positive responses to challenges all occurred between 5 min and 2 h of initiating the challenge. Symptoms associated with immediate response were distinctive and generally lasted 1–2 h. Several patients experienced increased cutaneous pruritus and transient morbilliform rash 6–10 h after the initial positive challenge. Symptoms associated with late response were less marked than those with immediate response and tended to last for several hours. No discernable isolated "delayed" reactions have been seen.

Many reports have suggested that children with atopic dermatitis are sensitive to a large number of food antigens. Although most children in this study had positive prick skin tests to several foods (mean, 3.2; range, 0–8), only about one-third of positive prick skin tests correlated with positive food challenges. In fact, most children (81%) reacted to only one or two foods by DBPCFC. Fifty-nine children (51%) reacted to only one food, 35 (30%) reacted to two foods, 18 (15%) reacted to three foods, and 5 children (4%) reacted to four or more different foods. Six food antigens - egg, peanut, milk, wheat, fish, and soy - accounted for about 90% of the positive clinical responses (Table 1).

Clinical reactivity to foods appears to be highly specific. Although results of skin tests (and RAST) commonly demonstrate cross-reactivity among members of a botanical family or animal species, there were only two cases of intrabotanical cross-reactivity and only one case of intraspecies cross-reactivity, as determined by DBPCFC. Consequently, the practice of avoiding all foods within a botanical family when one member of it is suspected of provoking allergic symptoms appears to be unwarranted.

Since patients experiencing positive DBPCFC developed a pruritic morbilliform rash instead of the classical urticarial lesion, markers of mast cell activation were sought. In a study of 33 patients undergoing DBPCFC [18], plasma histamine was measured prior to challenge and following ingestion of the test antigen. Patients ingesting placebo or a food which did not provoke clinical symptoms showed no demonstrable rise in their plasma histamine concentration. However, subjects experiencing clinical symptoms following the blind challenge devel-

Table 1. Foods eliciting hypersensitivity responses in 189 atopic dermatitis patients studied by DBPCFC

Antigen	Number of patients	Number positive[a]	Percent
Egg	90	5	41
Peanut	34	17	15
Milk	32	2	14
Soy	17	1	8
Fish	13	4	6
Wheat	9		4
Chicken	4		2
Beef	4	1	2
Pork	2		1
Potato	3	1	1
Others	14		6
Total	222		100

[a] Patients diagnosed on basis of "convincing" history (see text).

oped a rise in their plasma histamine (mean, from 296±80 pg/ml to 1055±356 pg/ml; $p<0.001$).

To determine whether basophils had been activated during the challenge and were contributing to the rise in plasma histamine, blood samples were obtained prior to challenge, immediately following, and 30 min following the development of the first objective symptoms [19]. Samples were evaluated for basophil number and total histamine content of the leukocyte preparation. There was no difference in basophil number or total histamine content at any time point. This suggests that circulating basophils do not contribute significantly to the observed changes in plasma histamine.

Several investigators have demonstrated the presence of circulating food-antigen–antibody complexes following oral food challenge [20–22]. To rule out complement activation of mast cells, a very sensitive radioimmunoassay was used to quantitate C3a des-Arg and C5a des-Arg prior to DBPCFC and immediately, 15 min, and 30 min following the development of objective symptoms. Measurement of the anaphylatoxins C3a and C5a is a very sensitive indicator of complement activation [23]. There was no significant change in plasma C3a des-Arg concentrations following positive DBPCFC in 18 patients. C5a des-Arg was not detectable in any samples examined. Therefore, it is extremely unlikely that complement-induced anaphylactoid reactions account for changes in plasma histamine following positive food challenges.

Results of the DBPCFC indicate that IgE-mediated food hypersensitivity readily produces a pruritic erythematous rash in some children with atopic dermatitis [17, 18, 24]. Symptoms that appear distinct when foods are ingested in isolation on an empty stomach during the DBPCFC appear less pronounced when the food is ingested at regular meals with other foods. Consequently, exacerbations of symptoms appear less distinct and blend into each other. Perhaps more central to the pathogenesis of atopic dermatitis, however, is the role of the "late phase" of IgE-mediated hypersensitivity.

Dolovich et al. [25] were first to describe the late-phase cutaneous allergic reaction (LCAR) in humans nearly 15 years ago. Solley and coworkers demonstrated that this reaction was dependent upon IgE [26]. Over 50 years ago, Walzer and his colleagues [27, 28] demonstrated unequivocally that ingested food antigens cross the gastrointestinal barrier and came into contact with skin mast cells fom within minutes to 2 h of ingestion. Although experimental forms of LCAR utilize allergens injected into the skin instead of those introduced via the circulation, they provide a useful model for studying mechanisms involved in cutaneous reactions secondary to food hypersensitivity.

Within minutes of encountering an allergen, cutaneous mast cells become activated and release histamine (and other mediators) into local tissue. This results in pruritus, vasodilation (seen as erythema), and capillary "leakiness" (seen as edema). Approximately 2–4 h later, neutrophils and eosinophils infiltrate the area. Once present, neutrophils could contribute to skin pathology by releasing various proinflammatory mediators: PGDs, LTB_4, PAF, and toxic oxygen radicals. Eosinophils, which may play a more prominent role in man, may release a variety of mediators which could contribute to pathogenesis [29, 30], as discussed below. Over the ensuing 24–48 h, monocytes and lymphocytes infiltrate the area, presenting a histologic picture indistinguishable from a type IV, cell-mediated response.

The paucity of eosinophils seen in histologic section of skin biopsies from eczematous lesions [16] cast doubt on the role of a late-phase mechanism in atopic dermatitis. However, in a study of LEIFERMAN et al. [31], biopsies from patients with atopic dermatitis were evaluated for the presence of eosinopohil major basic protein (MBP), a cytolytic protein secreted almost exclusively by eosinophils. Using an antibody specific for MBP and an indirect fluorescein-staining technique, specimens from 18 patients were examined. MBP was deposited in the superficial dermis of all specimens taken from eczematous skin lesions. MBP was not found in biopsy specimens from uninvolved skin sites in these same patients, indicating that this eosinophil product was the result of specific deposition and not of nonspecific sequestration via the circulation. Evaluation of biopsy specimens from other skin disorders, including contact dermatitis, did not reveal similar deposition of MBP.

More recently, two food-allergic patients, who had experienced clearing of their skin lesions after maintaining appropriate food-allergen restricted diets, underwent repeat DBPCFC in a subsequent study. Both patients developed a pruritic morbilliform skin rash within 30–60 min. Skin biopsy specimens obtained from involved sites 4 and 14 h later revealed an infiltration of eosinophils and MBP deposition. The dermal infiltrate contained more eosinophils and less prominent MBP deposition than was seen with the chronic lesions. These finding support the theory that food-allergen-induced mast cell activation can trigger both an immediate and a late-phase response in the skin. Furthermore, it suggests that the typical mononuclear round cell infiltrate found in atopic dermatitis skin lesions may result from an IgE-mediated mechanism.

The pathogenic role of eosinophils in eczematous skin lesions remains to be established. Earlier theories that eosionophil-associated enzymes dampen anaphylactic reactions by neutralizing many mediators of anaphylaxis - including histamine, slow-reacting substances of anaphylaxis, and platelet-activating factor - are doubted [29]. Besides MBP, eosinophils may release several other mediators which could contribute to the eczematous changes seen in skin biopsy specimens: eosinophil cationic protein (ECP), eosinophil-derived neurotoxin (EDN), and eosinophil peroxidase [29]. MBP is toxic to many cell types and can cause histamine release from mast cells [32, 33]. ECP, a potent neurotoxin, has been shown to inhibit lymphocyte proliferation and could contribute to the cutaneous anergy seen in patients with atopic dermatitis. EDN, also a powerful neurotoxin, may account for the demyelination of nerves in the dermal layer seen in eczematous skin.

Mechanisms other than direct food-antigen - antibody interaction may be involved in activation of cutaneous mast cells. One possibility is histamine-releasing factor (HRF), first described by Theuson and Grant et al. [34, 35]. Since their initial description, several investigators have identified HRFs from a variety of sources, including lymphocytes [36, 27], lung macrophages [38], and platelets [39]. These factors probably activate mast cells and basophils by binding to surface-bound IgE molecules [40]. Such factors may be responsible for chronic inflammation of the skin and for cutaneous hyperirritability.

In recent studies [19], patients with atopic dermatitis and food hypersensitivity were found to have high "spontaneous" histamine release (SBHR) from peripheral blood basophils in vitro (mean, 34% versus 2.6%; $p < 0.001$). In contrast, patients who had experienced good clearing of their skin lesions while maintaining the appropriate food-allergen avoidance diet for at least 1 year were found to have significantly lower SBHR (4.9% versus 34%; $p < 0.001$). In addition, peripheral blood mononuclear cells from food-allergic individuals were found to produce an HRF which could activate basophils from other food-sensitive individuals but not from food-nonsensitive subjects. HRF was synthesized in vitro even in mononuclear cells which had not been exposed to food allergen for several months. Ingestion of food antigens may lead to HRF production in vivo, which then could activate or lower the threshold of mast cell activation. It also could account for the increased basophil releasability seen in some patients with atopic dermatitis [41] and the high SBHR seen in food sensitive subjects in vitro.

IgE may effect a number of immunologic responses through non-mast cell IgE-mediated mechanisms. Low-affinity Fc_E receptors are found on B cells, T cells, monocytes, macrophages [42, 43], eosinophils [44], and platelets [45, 46]. Recently, BRUYNZEEL et al. [47] demonstrated that IgE molecules are bound to epidermal LCs only in patients with atopic dermatitis. The increased number of LCs in eczematous skin lesions and the frequent improvement in atopic dermatitis patients exposed to ultraviolet light (which selectively destroys LCs) suggest a central role for LCs in the pathogenesis of atopic dermatitis. It is therefore possible that food antigens or HRF may react with surface-bound IgE on several different cells capable of releasing a variety of inflammatory mediators.

The best method for diagnosing food hypersensitivity in children with atopic dermatitis remains controversial. Information generated in these studies strongly implicate IgE-mediated food hypersensitivity in the pathogenesis of atopic dermatitis. Unfortunately, the routine procedures of the allergist are not very useful in making the diagnosis. Historical information and elimination diets have rarely been helpful [17, 24]. Similarly, laboratory data are of limited value. Results of prick skin tests and RAST were of limited value in diagnosing food allergy [48]. The positive prick skin test was of only marginal value in identifying clinically relevant allergens. However, the negative prick skin test virtually excluded immediate food hypersensitivity in this disorder, unless presented with a convincing history to the contrary.

Therapy of IgE-mediated food hypersensitivity is straightforward. Strict avoidance of the offending food allergen is the only proven therapy. A recently completed double-blind placebo controlled cross-over trial of orally administered cromolyn sodium in 10 patients with atopic dermatitis and food hypersensitivity, proven by DBPCFC, demonstrated no benefit from this preparation [49]. Other therapeutic modalities that have been proposed, such as rotational diets, immunotherapy, sublingual neutralization, and subcutaneous neutralization, have never been shown to be efficacious in controlled trials.

Strict food-allergen avoidance may be required for only a few years, since clinical tolerance often develops. Approximately 1 year after initiating an appropriate elimination diet, 67 children with food hypersensitivity were rechallenged to 99 antigens. Overall, the 67 children studied developed clinical tolerance to one-third of the foods previously provoking an allergic response, although laboratory studies (prick skin tests and RAST) remained unchanged. Loss of food sensitivity varied somewhat depending upon the antigen in question. Patients allergic to peanut, wheat, egg, and milk were less likely to lose their sensitivity than children allergic to other food antigens.

To determine the significance of IgE-mediated food hypersensitivity in the pathogenesis of atopic dermatitis, the clinical courses of patients appropriately diagnosed and maintained on a relevant antigen-free diet were followed prospectively. Thirty-four children were followed for 3–4 years [24]: one group consisted of 17 children with food hypersensitivity who were maintained on appropriate elimination diets (food-sensitive group), and the other group comprised 12 children in whom no food hypersensitivity could be detected by DBPCFC and 5 children who were food sensitive but failed to comply with the diet (food-nonsensitive group). Cutaneous symptoms were scored at 6-month intervals using a standardized symptom score sheet. The scoring scale ranged from 0 (no symptoms) to 30 (severe symptoms) and was based on the patient's daytime and nighttime pruritus, extent of skin rash, medication requirements (antihistamines, antibiotics, and corticosteroids), physician visits, and days absent from school. Total serum IgE concentrations were compared since they have been shown to correlate with disease severity in atopic dermatitis [50, 51]. There was no significant difference between the two groups in symptom scores or serum IgE concentrations at the initiation of the study. However, the food-sensitive group showed a highly significant improvement in their clinical scores by midstudy (median, from 21 to 8; $p<0.001$) with further slight improvement by the end of the study period (median, 6). The food-nonsensitive group experienced slight improvement in their clinical score by midstudy (median, from 20 to 17; $p<0.05$) which remained unchanged through the remainder of the study (median, 17). The slight improvement that was seen was probably due to more intensive skin care, since the improvement occurred early and did not change over the course of the study. The clinical symptom scores of the food-sensitive group were significantly better than those of the nonsensitive group at midstudy and at the end of the study period (8 versus 17; $p<0.001$). The food-sensitive group experienced a significant decrease in total IgE over the course of the study (midstudy, $p=0.045$; poststudy, $p=0.037$) whereas the food-nonsensitive group experienced an increase in total serum IgE values. The five patients with food hypersensitivity in the food-nonsensitive group showed no significant improvement in their clinical course (median prestudy, 20; midstudy, 19; final, 20), and all experienced an increase in their total serum IgE concentration over the course of the study. These data support the claim that appropriate diagnosis and elimination of foods provoking hypersensitivity responses favorably affect the course of atopic dermatitis.

Although considerable controversy continues over the prophylactic role of breast feeding, the weight of recent evidence sugests a beneficial effect in the prevention (or at least postponement) of allergic disorders. In one study by SAARINEN et al. [52], exclusive breast feeding was found to reduce the number of infants developing food hypersensitivity and atopic dermatitis in the 1st year of life. However, further follow-up suggested that breast feeding may simply postpone the development of atopic disease in those predisposed infants not developing clinical hypersensitivity in the 1st year [53]. Since breast feeding provides many other benefits to the developing infant, even postponing food allergy until after the neonatal period is in itself sufficient reason to advocate this practice.

The studies reported here demonstrate a significant role for IgE-mediated reactions to foods in the pathogenesis of atopic dermatitis in at least some patients. Mechanisms involved in the pathogenesis of the eczematous rash may incorporate IgE molecules in hypersensitivity reactions other than the classic Gell and Coombs type I, immediate hypersensitivity response. More research obviously will be necessary to clarify this issue.

References

1. Blaylock WK (1976) Atopic dermatitis: diagnosis and pathobiology. J Allergy Clin Immunol 57:62-79
2. Hill LW, Sulzberger MG (1935) Evaluation of atopic dermatitis. Arch Belg Dermatol Syphiligr 32:451-463
3. Hanifin JM, Rajka G (1980) Diagnostic features of atopic dermatitis. Acta Derm Venerol 92 (Suppl):44-47
4. Hanifin JM (1981) Atopic dermatitis. In: Safari B, Good RA (eds) Comprehensive immunology. Plenum, New York, p 301
5. Wise F, Sulzberger MB (1983) Yearbook of dermatology and syphilology. Yearbook Medical, Chicago, p 59
6. Johnson ML (1977) Prevalence of dermatologic disease among persons 1-74 years of age: United States. Advance data from vital and health statistics of the National Center for Health Statistics, no 4
7. Kjellman N-IM (1977) Atopic disease in seven year old children. Acta Paediatr Scand 66:465-71
8. Hanifin JM (1986) Pharmacophysiology of atopic dermatitis. Clin Rev Allergy 4:43-65
9. Leung DYM, Geha RS (1986) Immunoregulatory abnormalities in atopic dermatitis. Clin Rev Allergy 4:67-86
10. NIAID Task Force Report (1979) Dermatologic allergy. Asthma and the other allergic diseases. NIH Publication no 79-387, (1974) p 375
11. Johnson E, Irons J, Patterson R, Roberts M (1974) Serum IgE concentration in atopic dermatitis. J Allergy Clin Immunol 54:94-99

12. Rajka G (1975) The Aetiology of atopic dermatitis. In: Rook A (ed) Major problems in dermatology. Atopic dermatitis, vol 3. Saunders, London, pp 52–54
13. Hofman DR, Yamamoto FY, Sellar B, Haddad Z (1975) Diagnosis of IgE-mediated reactions to food antigens by radioimmunoassay. Clin Immunol 55:256–267
14. Pasternack B (1965) The prediction of asthma in infantile eczema. J Pediatr 66:164–165
15. Stifler WC (1965) A twenty-one year follow-up of infantile eczema. J Pediatr 66:166–167
16. Mihm MC, Soter NA, Dvorak HF, Austen KF (1976) The structure of normal skin and the morphology of atopic eczema. J Invest Dermatol 67:305–312
17. Sampson HA (1985) Role of immediate food hypersensitivity in the pathogenesis of atopic dermatitis. J Allergy Clin Immunol 71:473–478
18. Sampson HA, Jolie PA (1984) Increased plasma histamine concentrations after food challenges in children with atopic dermatitis. N Engl J Med 311:372–376
19. Sampson HA, Broadbent K (1987) "Spontaneous" basophil histamine release and histamine releasing factor in patients with atopic dermatitis and food hypersensitivity. J Allergy Clin Immunol 79:241
20. Paganelli R, Levinsky RJ, Brostoff J, Wraith DG (1979) Immune complexes containing food proteins in normal and atopic subjects after oral challenge and effect of sodium cromoglycate on antigen absorption. Lancet 1:1270
21. Brostoff J, Carini C, Wraith DG, Johns P (1979) Production of IgE complexes by allergen challenge in atopic patients and the effect of sodium cromoglycate. Lancet 1:1268
22. Paganelli R, Atherton DJ, Levinsky R (1983) Differences between normal and milk allergic subjects in their immune responses after milk ingestion. Arch Dis Child 58:201
23. Chenowith DE, Hugli TE (1980) Biologically active peptides of complement: techniques and significance of C3a and C5a measurement. In: Nakamura RM, Tucker ES (eds) Immunoassays: clinical laboratory techniques for the 1980's.Liss, New York, pp 443–461
24. Sampson HA, McCaskill CM (1985) Food hypersensitivity in atopic dermatitis: evaluation of 113 patients. J Pediatr 107:669
25. Dolovich J, Hargreave FE, Chalmers R, Shier KJ, Gauldre J, Bienenstock J (1973) Late cutaneous allergic responses in isolated IgE-dependent reactions. J Allergy Clin Immunol 52:38
26. Solley GO, Gleich GJ, Jordan RE, Schroeter AL (1976) The late phase of the immediate wheal and flare skin reaction: its dependence upon IgE antibodies. J Clin Invest 58:408
27. Brunner M, Walzer M (1928) Absorption of undigested proteins in human beings: the absorption of unaltered fish protein in adults. Arch Intern Med 42:173
28. Wilson SJ, Walzer M (1935) Absorption of undigested proteins in human beings. IV. Absorption of unaltered egg protein in infants. Am J Dis Child 50:49
29. Gleich GJ, Leiferman KM (1986) Eosinophils and hypersensitivity disease. In: Reed CE (ed) Proceedings of the XII International Congress of Allergology and Clinical Immunology. Mosby, St. Louis, pp 124–130
30. Leiferman KM, Peters MS, Gleich GJ (1986) The eosinophil and cutaneous edema. J Am Acad Dermatol 15:513

31. Leiferman KM, Ackerman SJ, Sampson HA, Haugen HS, Venenice PY, Gleich GJ (1985) Dermal deposition of eosinophil granule major basic protein in atopic dermatitis: comparison with onchocerciasis. N Engl Med 313:282–285
32. Gleich GJ, Frigas E, Loegering DA, Wassom DL, Steinmuller D (1979) Cytotoxic properties of eosinophil major basic protein. J Immunol 123:2925–2927
33. O'Donnel MC, Ackerman SJ, Gleich GJ, Thomas LL (1983) Activation of basophil and mast cell histamine release by eosinophil granule major basic protein. J Exp Med 157:1981–1991
34. Thueson DO, Speck LS, Lett-Brown MA, Grant JA (1979) Histamine-releasing activity. I. Production by mitogen- or antigen-stimulated human mononuclear cells. J Immunol 123:626
35. Thueson DO, Speck LS, Lett-Brown MA, Grant JA (1979) Histamine-releasing activity. II. Interaction with basopohils and physicochemical characterization. J Immunol 123:633
36. Sedgwick JD, Holt PG, Turner KJ (1981) Production of a histamine-releasing lymphokine by antigen- or mitogen-stimulated human peripheral T cells. Clin Exp Immunol 45:409
37. Kaplan AP, Haak-Frendscho M, Fauci A, Dinarello, Halbert E (1985) A histamine-releasing factor from activated human mononuclear cells. J Immunol 135:2027
38. Schulman ES, Proud D, Liu MC, MacGlashan DW, Lichtenstein LM, Plaut M (1985) Human lung macrophages induce histamine release from basophils and mast cells. Am Rev Respir Dis 131:230
39. Orchard MA, Kagey-Sobotka A, Proud D, Lichtenstein LM (1986) Basophil histamine release induced by a substance from stimulated human platelets. J Immunol 136:2240
40. McDonald SM, Lichtenstein LM, Proud D, Plaut M, Naclerio RM, MacGlashan DW, Kagey-Sobotka A (1987) Studies of IgE-dependent histamine releasing factors: heterogeneity of IgE. J Immunol 139:506
41. Marone G, Giugliano R, Lembo G, Ayala F (1986) Human basophil releasability. II. Changes in basopohil releasability in patients with atopic dermatitis. J Invest Dermatol 87:19
42. Yodoi J, Ishizaka K (1979) Lymphocytes bearing Fc-receptors for IgE. 1. Presence of human and rat lymphocytes with Fc_E-receptors. J Immunol 122:2577
43. Spiegelberg HL (1984) Structure and function of Fc receptors for IgE on lymphocytes, monocytes and macrophages. Adv Immunol 35:61
44. Capron M, Spiegelberg HL, Prin L, Bennich H, Butterworth AE, Pierce RJ, Ouaissi M, Capron A (1984) Role of IgE receptors in effector function of human eosinophils. J Immunol 132:462
45. Capron A, Ameisen JC, Joseph M, Auriault C, Tonnel AB, Caen J (1985) New functions for platelets and their pathological implications. Int Arch Allergy Appl Immunol 77:107
46. Cines DB, van der Keyl H, Levinson AI (1986) In vitro binding of an IgE protein to human platelets. J Immunol 136:3433
47. Bruynzeel-Koomen C, van Wichen DF, Toonstra J, Berrens L, Bruynzeel PLB (1986) The presence of IgE molecules on epidermal Langerhans cells in patients with atopic dermatitis. Arch Dermatol Res 278:199
48. Sampson HA, Albergo R (1984) Comparison of results of skin tests, RAST, and double-blind placebo-controlled food challenges in children with atopic dermatitis. J Allergy Clin Immunol 74:26–33

49. Burks AW, Sampson HA (1988) A controlled trial of oral cromolyn in children with atopic dermatitis and documented food hypersensitivity. J Allergy Clin Immunol 81:417–423
50. Ohman S, Johansson SGO (1974) Immunoglobulins in atopic dermatitis. Acta Derm Venerol 54:193–202
51. Stone SP, Gleich GJ, Muller SA (1976) Atopic dermatitis and IgE relationship between changes in IgE levels and severity of disease. Arch Dermatol 112:1254–1255
52. Kajosaari M, Saarinen UM (1983) Prophylaxis of atopic disease by six months total solid food elimination. Acta Paediatr Scand 72:411
53. Saarinen UM, Kajosaari M (1980) Does dietary elimination in infancy prevent or only postpone a food allergy? Lancet 1:166

Food Allergy and Asthma

J. Bousquet and F. B. Michel

Food allergy has always been a difficult problem, especially in asthma, where some investigators deny its existence while others tend to overestimate its role. The difficulties stem not only from the concept that ingested allergens may not be able to trigger mast cells present in the airways but also from the diagnosis of food allergy, which is often less than accurate [5].

There are several cases demonstrating that asthma can be triggered by foods, and that an appropriate diet is able to control asthma. However, many clinical cases are only speculative, and it is always extremely difficult to ascribe an asthma attack to food allergy when the delay between ingestion and symptoms exceeds 24 h, owing to the great variability in types of airway obstruction in chronic asthmatics. Here we present some demonstrative cases of food allergy in asthmatic children and adults.

Diagnosis of Food Allergy Inducing Asthma

The diagnosis of food allergy is difficult because allergen extracts currently available are not standardized, and their stability is poorly determined. For allergen extracts that are rapidly degraded, such as those of fruits and legumes, skin tests may be falsely negative in food-allergic individuals. Conversely, some extracts contain irritative and mast cell degranulating substances which cause false-positive skin tests. The titration of serum food-specific IgE is available only for certain foods, and in contrast to better characterized inhalant allergens the sensitivity of the test is not yet fully known for most unpurified food allergens. Moreover, even more so than in the case of inhalant allergy, the presence of food IgE in serum or of positive skin tests to foods do not always correlate with a food allergy since (a) many patients outgrow their allergy with age, (b) not all patients with IgE have a clinical sensitivity [9].

Patients who develop acute urticaria or anaphylaxis often make the diagnosis of food intolerance by themselves, and the presence of positive skin tests and/or serum specific IgE correlating with the claims of the patient makes possible a diagnosis without performing a food challenge. This test may cause severe untoward reactions in patients with anaphylaxis and should not be done. However, in asthma, patients rarely incriminate a food as the cause of wheezing; in this case the clinician must suspect a food allergy and confirm the diagnosis by double-blind food challenges [1].

Food allergy should be suspected in the following cases: (a) when asthma started early in life, especially if the patient has had or currently presents atopic dermatitis; (b) when total serum IgE is over 1000 IU/l by the paper radioimmunosorbent test (PRIST); (c) in patients presenting anaphylactic symptoms or acute urticaria due to food allergy; and (d) in any patient, even in adults, with poorly controlled asthma and elevated total serum IgE levels. In our experience, patients with gastrointestinal tract (GIT) symptoms do not present food allergy more often than those without GIT symptoms. Suspicion of food allergy does not mean diagnosis of food allergy.

In our clinic all asthmatic patients, regardless of age, undergo screnning for food allergy by means of prick tests to the seven most common foods of the area. Patients in whom food allergy is suspected have a comlete screening for food allergens by prick tests. When a prick test is positive, serum specific IgE to the given food is titrated. In patients having clear symptoms with certain foods but in whom skin prick tests are negative, a screening of serum specific IgE is done. The presence of positive skin prick test and/or serum specific IgE does not preclude the positivity of a food challenge, since only one-third of patients presenting with positive skin prick tests and/or serum specific IgE have asthma during food challenge, so that a diet should not be started before food challenges have been performed. Some investigators use intradermal skin tests, but, although they may detect IgG short-term sensitizing (STS) and have been shown to be slightly more sensitive than skin prick tests, they also cause more nonspecific positive reactions and may induce systemic reactions. The presence of a positive skin test is indicative for a food challenge.

The titration of serum food-specific IgG or IgG4 may be done, however one must note that (a) it is not certain that such antibodies are present in greater amounts in food-allergic patients, since they may be present in the serum of totally healthy individuals, and (b) they do not mean more than serum specific IgE or skin tests. Food challenges must therefore confirm the diagnosis of asthma due to food allergy.

Food challenges should be performed in a manner similar to that reported by Bock and May [1] or Sampson and Albergo [7]. The food suspected of causing symptoms should be eliminated from the diet for a minimum of 2 weeks before testing. The selection of foods for administration is based upon positive skin tests and/or specific IgE or on a strongly positive history despite negative skin prick tests and/or radio-allergosorbent tests (RAST). Patients should stop medications that might modify the performance of the test for an appropriate delay. When possible, lyophilized foods should be placed in size 0 dye-free opaque capsules, or, if administered as a liquid, they should be mixed in a broth or a juice to disguise the taste. Although patients who present anaphylactic symptoms should not be tested, it is advised to increase the doses slowly from 100 mg to 10 g. Challenges should, at best, be done in a double-blind manner, but if several foods are incriminated, a screening with single-blind challenges may be done first. In case of food-induced asthma, pulmonary function tests should be done serially for up to 8 h since late reactions may occur. During the entire challenge a physician should follow up the patient since some untoward systemic reaction may occur. The challenge is considered positive only if $PD_{20}FEV_1$ is reached on test day without any such drop in FEV_1 during placebo day. In young children, pulmonary function tests are not easy to perform and to interprete without sophisticated equipment that is not always available; the diagnosis of asthma may therefore be based only on clinical examination. Some patients develop GIT symptoms, acute urticaria, or atopic dermatitis without any airway response. A positive food challenge does not necessarily imply that the patient presents an IgE-mediated allergy, but merely that he is intolerant to the foods. If specific IgE and/or prick tests to this food are positive, an IgE-mediated mechanism is likely to be involved. When oral cromoglycate is commercially available, a further food challenge may be done to test the efficacy of this drug in the patient in order to propose such a treatment [6].

Elimination diets are used primarily for the diagnosis of chronic diseases, such as eczema and rhinitis. In the case of asthma, it is often difficult to make the diagnosis of food allergy by elimination diets for many reasons. (a) Food allergy is often associated with inhalant allergy and possibly with other triggers, and variations in airway obstruction may be due to factors unrelated to foods. (b) Food allergens as well as inhalant allergens aggravate nonspecific bronchial hyperreactivity, and it may take days or even weeks to observe an improvement of asthma. (c) The great variability of airway obstruction in chronic asthmatics may shadow the benefits of dietary manipulations. However, when a patient is highly allergic to a given food, significant improvement or even complete remission of asthma can be observed.

As for other forms of food allergy, unproven and controversial techniques such as cytotoxic tests or sublingual provocation tests have absolutely to value.

Incidence of Food Allergy in Asthma

Asthma due to foods may be related either to IgE-mediated food allergy, IgG-mediated food allergy, or to intolerance to various compounds, including sulfites, dyes, and other preservatives. IgE-mediated allergy appears to be much less common than food intolerance as a trigger of asthma. At present there is no definitive proof that IgG or IgG4 are important immunoglobulin isotypes in food allergy, or that they can induce exacerbations of asthma days after the food intake. More data are thus needed to clarify this problem. Finally, activated lymphocytes may also be involved in food allergy, but this is only speculative [4].

Although some investigators have proposed that many, if not most, so-called intrinsic asthmatics are in fact allergic to foods [8], the few controlled studies available do not substantiate this assertion. In areas where mugwort and birch pollens are rare, food allergy represents only a minor cause of asthma. Moreover, food allergy is often associated with inhalant allergy. We have observed that only 3%–5% of asthmatic children have bronchial symptoms in which food allergy is implicated. In adults the percentage is even smaller and does not exceed 1%. However, in areas where mugwort and birch pollens are prevalent, allergy due to cross-reactive foods, such as celery or fruits, may be more important, but anaphylactic, or gastrointestinal and dermatological symptoms are likely to be more frequent than asthma [2]. Finally, differences may be observed due to specific features of the usual diet of a given country.

Treatment of Asthma Induced by Food Allergy

The presence of a positive skin prick test or RAST to a given food should not lead to an elimination diet because only 30%–40% of patients have asthma when they are challenged orally with the offending food. This finding was already observed for atopic dermatitis and other food-induced symptoms except anaphylaxis. In case of a positive food challenge, dietary avoidance should be started, but denutrition must always be avoided especially in young children [3].

Oral cromoglycate was found in some, but not all, studies to prevent asthma due to food allergy. It is clear that only a fraction of patients benefit from this treatment, but, when available and effective, it may be used (a) to decrease the reactivity of the GIT to dietary allergens and (b) to allow a less restrictive diet. Ketotifene was also used and seemed to have a greater value in the treatment of skin symptoms, whereas this drug is also used in the treatment of food-asthma.

There is at present no evidence to support specific immunotherapy by either the oral or the parenteral route.

In any case, asthma is a disease of the airways, and patients should always receive treatment for bronchial inflammation and obstruction in addition to that for food allergy.

References

1. Bock SA, May CD (1983) Adverse reactions to food caused by sensitivity. In: Middleton E Jr, Reed CE, Ellis EF (eds) Allergy, principles and practice. Mosby, St Louis, p 1415
2. Eriksson NE (1978) Food sensitivity reported by patients with asthma and hay fever. Allergy 33:189
3. Ganderton MA (1978) Diet and asthma. Br Med J i:1624
4. Lessof MH (1983) Reactions to foods in adults. In: Lessof MH (ed) Clinical reactions to foods. Wiley, London, p 103
5. Metcalfe D (1984) Food hypersensitivity. J Allergy Clin Immunol 73:749
6. Onorato J, Merland N, Terral C, Michel FB, Bousquet J (1986) Placebo-controlled double-blind food challenge. J Allergy Clin Immunol 78:1139
7. Sampson HA, Albergo R (1984) Comparison of results of skin tests, RAST and double-blind, placebo-controlled food challenges in children with atopic dermatitis. J Allergy Clin Immunol (1982) 75:348
8. Wraith DG (1982) Asthma. Clin Immunol Allergy 2:101
9. Committee on Adverse Reactions to Food (1984) Adverse reactions to food. American Academy of Allergy and Immunology. National Institute of Allergy and Infections Disease, Besthesda

Food Allergy and Disorders of the Central Nervous System in Childhood

J. Egger

Introduction

Interactions between psyche and soma are complex, and nowhere is this better demonstrated than in patients with multiple food allergies. In these patients psychosomatic and somatopsychic influences sometimes interact to such an extent that without systematic controlled provocation studies it would be impossible to accept a causative role for foods at all.

The idea that what one eats influences how one feels and behaves is not new. Some 2000 years ago TITUS LUCRETIUS CARUS coined the saying, "One man's meat is another man's poison". In the seventeenth century RICHARD BURTON proclaimed in the "Anatomy of Melancholy" that milk, and all that comes from it, increases melancholy. Early this century a comprehensive monograph was published on associations between food allergy and various symptoms of the central nervous system (CNS) [62], to which little could be added to date.

Links between the ingestion of food and symptoms of the CNS may arise in a variety of ways, many of which are probably not yet known. The following definitions can be used for practical purposes, however different types of reactions to foods may not only occur singly but also in any combination.

1. *Food intolerance.* This is a reproducible physical and/or psychological reaction to food, occurring independently of a person's awareness of the nature of the food ingested. It may occur for a variety of reasons, such as allergy, enzyme defects, pharmacological action, histamine release, reactions to toxic substances (e.g. lead), and for reasons as yet unascertained.
2. *Psychologically based reactions to food.* These are reactions that depend on the person's awareness of the nature of the food ingested.

3. *Food avoidance*. This is a form of behaviour involving deliberate abstention from foods for whatever reasons, e.g. religion, anorexia nervosa, and dieting.

Studies using double-blind procedures have established that foods are relevant in causing a number of chronic disorders of the CNS [29–31] however the nature of the causal link between foods and symptoms is not yet understood.

Migraine

The cause of migraine is not known. Perhaps migraine is best regarded as a neurovascular syndrome with a generalized vasomotor instability and vulnerability to multiple factors. The apparent precipitating factors may be the final event leading to decompensation of the system. These include the following:

- Emotional factors
- Food
- Trauma
- Exertion
- Upper respiratory tract infection
- Hypoglycaemia
- Lactose intolerance
- Irregular sleep
- Weather changes
- Travel
- Bright light
- Noise
- Hormonal factors

Whether food intolerance is but one of the precipitating factors or whether it causes the neurovascular instability cannot be answered at present.

Publications concerning the relationship between migraine and dietary factors can be separated into two groups, according to whether they support the tyramine hypothesis or the food allergy hypothesis.

Tyramine Hypothesis. HANNINGTON [41] reported that foods containing tyramine or other vasoactive amines may precipitate headaches, particularly in patients who are treated with monoamino-oxidase inhibitors. A defect in the conjugation of tyramine phenylaethylamine was incriminated by some authors [65] and others proposed a deficiency of platelete phenolsulphotransferase [46], but double-blind administration of tyramine to patients who seemed to be affected in this way did not provoke migraine [16].

Food Allergy Hypothesis. There are multiple case reports in the older literature of migraine attacks which have been associated with severe generalized allergic reactions to foods [9, 39, 47, 52, 53, 56, 63, 68, 71, 77]. Although most were purely anecdotal and are now regarded as impressionistic and unscientific, there is good evidence to incriminate food allergy in children with severe migraine [29]. However, it does not appear that this is due to central involvement of allergic mechanisms but rather to an influence on the permeability of the gut allowing increased ingress of vasoactive substances.

The Oligoantigenic Approach. All foods are potential allergens, and an oligoantigenic diet should contain as few foods as possible. An example of an oligoantigenic diet is the following:

- Lamb, turkey
- Potatoes, rice
- Pears, bananas
- Brassicas
- Sunflower oil
- Water, mineral water
- Calcium, vitamines

Sometimes the foods chosen may be provoking ones, and if there is no improvement or deterioration, an alternative oligoantigenic diet avoiding foods included in the first diet should be tried. If recovery or definite improvement occurs during 3–4 weeks of oligoantigenic diet treatment, other foods are reintroduced one-by-one at weekly intervals. If symptoms occur reproducibly with a certain food, it is withdrawn and eventually tested in a double-blind placebo-controlled crossover study [13]. The values of an oligoantigenic diet was demonstrated by a such trial [29] in which 93% of children with severe and frequent migraine (more than one per week) were shown to benefit. During the sequential reintroduction of foods at weekly intervals, 90% of the responders relapsed with one or more foods (Table 1) and recovered again avoiding

Table 1. Provoking foods in migraine ($n=76$)

Food	Number tested	Number reacted	Percent
Cow's milk	75	29	39
Chocolate	64	24	37
Benzoic acid	46	17	37
Eggs	71	26	36
Tartrazine	45	15	33
Wheat	71	22	31
Cheese	48	15	31
Citrus	72	22	30
Coffee	21	5	24
Fish	51	11	22
Maize	53	9	17
Grapes	23	4	17
Goat's milk	44	7	16
Tee	44	7	16
Pork	60	8	13
Beef	64	8	12
Beans	42	9	12
Malt	33	3	9
Lentils	21	2	9
Apples	74	6	8
Yeast	54	4	7
Pears	69	4	6
Apricote	48	3	6
Sugar	56	3	5
Potatoes	78	4	5
Peas	37	2	5
Banana	78	4	5
Carrots	76	3	4
Chicken	73	3	4
Peaches	51	2	4
Lamb	75	2	3
Rice	75	9	1
Brassica	76	1	1

From Egger et al. [29]

them. The interval between eating a provoking food and migraine varied from minutes to more then a week but was usually 2–3 days. A total of 46 children in whom provoking food was identified entered a double-blind placebo-controlled crossover trial of the provoking food, and highly significantly more patients had headaches with active material ($p<0.001$) than with placebo (Table 2).

Table 2. Results of a double-blind placebo-controlled crossover trial

Occurence of headaches with	A/P	P/A	Both
Neither food	2	6	8
Active food	14	12	26
Placebo	0	2	2
Both foods	1	3	4
Total	17	23	40

A, active material; P, placebo.
A/P versus P/A, NS; A versus P, $p < 0.001$.
From Egger et al. [29]

Table 3. Conners' abbreviated rating scales

Observation	Degree of activity			
	Not at all	Just a little	Pretty much	Very much
Restless or overactive				
Excitable, impulsive				
Disturbs other children				
Fails to finish things				
Short attention span				
Constantly fidgeting				
Inattentive, easily distracted				
Demands must be met immediately				
Easily frustrated				
Cries often and easily				
Mood changes quickly and drastically				
Temper outbursts				
Explosive and unpredictable behaviour				
Scoring	0	1	2	3

The Hyperkinetic Syndrome

Hyperkinetic behaviour is defined by overactivity, impulsivity, distractability and excitability. There is no standard of what is a normal level of activity on which to base comparisons, and the threshold for viewing such behaviour as pathological, or as a specific syndrome, varies very markedly between countries, between parents and between different physicians. So far, reliable and valid tests of overactivity are not available. For practical purposes behaviour rating scales are used, such as that of CONNERS [17] (Table 3); classification is by the criteria of the Diagnostic and Statistical Manual III [4]. Many causes of overactivity have been proposed. Suspected causes of overactivity include the following:

- Inherited hyperkinetic syndrome
- Adverse psychosocial situations
- Perinatal problems
- Brain damage
- Brain dysfunction
- Epilepsy
- Anticonvulsants
- Lead poisoning
- Maternal smoking during pregnancy
- Maternal alcohol intake during pregnancy
- Maternal drug abuse or drug intake during pregnancy
- Atopy
- Hypersensitivity to salicylates and synthetic food additives
- Food allergy
- Malnutrition
- Metabolic disorders
- Syndromes
- Chromosomal abnormalities

More than 92 terms have been used to describe hyperactive children, of which the commonest are "attention deficit disorder", "minimal brain dysfunction" and "hyperkinetic syndrome".

A number of treatments have been used, of which psychostimulant drugs [35], behavioural approaches [58] and diets are the commonest. Concern about the undesirable effects of drug treatment as well as the mounting evidence for the lack of long-term efficacy both of drug treatment and behavioural methods has led to a focus on diets. The diets tested in double-blind controlled trials were FEINGOLD's diet [18, 42, 73, 76, 82, 84], HAFER's phosphate-reduced diet [80], and oligoantigenic diets [30].

The Feingold Hypothesis. In June 1975 a preliminary report was presented by FEINGOLD [34], in which it was proposed that hyperkinesis in childhood is associated with the ingestion of salicylates, food additives and colours. FEINGOLD treated hyperactive children with diets avoiding all food additives as well as natural salicylates and claimed success in 70% of them. The report of his findings was impressionistic, anecdotal and lacking in objective evidence. Subsequently a number of double-blind trials involving control diets and diets eliminating artificial colours, flavours and salicylates were conducted on children with well-defined hyperkinetic syndrome [18, 42, 73, 76, 82, 84]. The results of these controlled studies of FEINGOLD's hypothesis are all somewhat equivocal, but their broad conclusions are that FEINGOLD's claims where probably exaggerated. The reason for the uncertainty is the lack of comparability between studies because of the heterogeneity of patients studied and differences in dietary manipulations. Moreover, research designs were inadequate. For example, control diets were used whose effects on behaviour had not studied [18, 42]. No washout periods were inserted between the distinct test periods, and these were probably disturbed by carry-over effects [42, 73, 76, 82, 84]. Active and placebo materials were disguised in chocolate and sugar-containing materials [73, 76, 84], although it is known that these substances are likely to have adverse effects on behaviour [30]. And the challanges were administered for only 1 or 2 days [73, 82], thus not allowing the symptoms to develop. However, all studies showed that some hyperactive children, or certain subgroups of them, may benefit from an additive-free diet.

The Phosphate Hypothesis. According to HAFER [40] phosphate is thought to play a major role in causing the hyperkinetic syndrome. Again, her evidence was purely anecdotal, and a controlled study on 35 children did not show a reproducible effect of the phosphate [80]. However, children on a phosphate-reduced diet would avoid many foods, including cow's milk, chocolate and foods containing artificial colors and preservatives, and it is not unlikely that children occasionally improve on it.

The Food Allergy Hypothesis. A role for food allergy in the hyperkinetic syndrome has been postulated since early this century [19, 21, 43, 59, 61, 63, 71]. Because of the lack of scientific documentation, this hypothesis was rejected until the highly significant results of a double-blind placebo-controlled crossover trial were published [30]. Of the 76 children who took part in this experiment, all were socially handicapped by their behaviour, and overactivity and inattention were prominent features.

Table 4. Provoking foods in patients with hyperkinetic syndrome ($n=62$)

Food	Tested	Symptoms	Percent
Colourant, preservatives	34	27	79
Soya	15	11	73
Cow's milk	55	35	64
Chocolate	34	20	59
Grapes	18	9	50
Wheat	53	28	49
Oranges	49	22	45
Cow's cheese	15	6	40
Hen's eggs	50	20	39
Peanuts	19	6	32
Maize	38	11	29
Fish	48	11	23
Oats	43	10	23
Melons	29	6	21
Tomatoes	35	7	20
Ham, bacon	20	4	20
Pineapple	31	6	19
Sugar	55	9	16
Beef	49	8	16
Beans	34	5	15
Peas	33	5	15
Malt	20	3	15
Apples	53	7	13
Pork	38	5	13
Pears	41	5	12
Chicken	56	6	11
Potatoes	54	6	11
Tea	19	2	10
Coffee	10	1	10
Other nuts	11	1	10
Cucumbers	32	3	9
Bananas	52	4	8
Carrots	55	4	7
Peaches	41	3	7
Lamb	55	3	5
Turkey	22	1	5
Rice	51	2	4
Yeast	28	1	4
Apricots	34	1	3
Onions	49	1	2

From Egger et al. [30]

The children were selected for severe overactivity and may not be representative of hyperkinetic children in the general population. A surprisingly high proportion had associated symptoms such as recurrent headaches, abdominal pains, limb pains and epileptic seizures, and only ten did not have any associated symptoms. Of all the children, 82% responded to an oligoantigenic diet. However, only 72% recovered completely. Most of the associated symptoms also improved with diet. During the subsequent reintroduction, the commonest substances that caused problems were tartrazine and benzoic acid, but no child reacted to these alone. Forty-six other provocative foods were also identified (Table 4), and most patients reacted reproducibly to several (Table 5). The interval between eating a provoking food and reaction was usually 2–3 days but varied from a few minutes to more than 7 days. There was no difference in type of reaction and length of the interval between eating the provoking item and appearance of symptoms between synthetic additives and foods.

Altogether, 28 patients completed the double-blind placebo-controlled crossover trial on the effect of reintroduction of a provoking food. The parents kept daily Conners' scores and a paediatrician and a child psychologist independently made an assessment of the children's behaviour for each arm of the double-blind trial. The psychologist also employed actometer readings, matching familiar-figures tests and the

Table 5. Number of foods to which patients reacted

Number of foods	Number of patients
1	5
2	4
3	4
4	8
5	4
6	9
7	3
8	4
9	3
10	3
11	2
12	2
18	1
21	1
27	1
30	2

Porteus-Maze test. Parents, the paediatrician and the psychologist assessed the period in which the placebo material was administered as being linked significantly more often with better behaviour (Table 6).

Follow-Up of Patients with Food Intolerance and Hyperkinetic Behaviour. Some of patients do not react to the provoking food when they are tested again after avoiding it for a period from 6 months to 1 year. On the other hand, foods previously shown not to cause problems sometimes (usually after viral infections) start to provoke symptoms and must be avoided.

Prognosis of the Hyperkinetic Syndrome. Early investigators thought that the hyperkinetic syndrome was a time-limited condition disappearing after adolescence. It is now recognized that, although hyperactivity may diminish with age, antisocial behaviour, educational retardation, depression and psychosis are prevalent in grown-up hyperkinetic children [50, 51, 83]. It is too early to speculate whether dietary management would influence the prognosis of hyperkinetic children. However, there are reports suggesting that antisocial behaviour in young delinquents is often related to certain foods and food additives [66], and that schizophrenics on a milk- and cereal-free diet were released from hospital twice as early as those given the regular hospital diet [28].

Table 6. Results of a double-blind placebo-controlled crossover trial

Behaviour better on	Paediatrician			Parents			Psychologist		
	P/A	A/P	Both	P/A	A/P	Both	A/P	P/A	Both
Neither	3	4	7	2	2	4	5	4	9
Placebo	12	8	20	13	10	23	7	6	13
Active	0	1	1	0	1	1	0	2	2
Total	15	13	28	15	13	28	12	12	24

PA v AP, NS; A v P <0.001
A, Active material; P, placebo
From Egger et al. [30]

Epilepsy

Throughout this century a possible provocation of seizures by foods or other allergens has been variously reported [10, 20, 23, 29, 30, 71, 75]. Some other clinical studies of epileptics found an unusually high prevalence of allergic disorders [2, 12, 22, 24, 25, 70, 79, 81], whereas an increased prevalence of electroencephalographic abnormalities often with occipital dysrhythmias was present in patients with allergic disorders [7, 11, 15, 24–26, 36, 72, 74]. However, others have not found an association between allergy and epilepsy [33], and the majority of reports on foods and seizures are anecdotal and open to alternative hypotheses. An exception is the study with double-blind placebo-controlled provocations in only one patient by CRAYTON et al. [20] and the double-blind placebo-controlled provocation studies in 16 children with epilepsy who had undergone oligoantigenic diet treatment for migraine and/or hyperkinetic behaviour [29, 30]. The results of these studies show clearly that some patients with epilepsy recover upon avoiding certain foods. However a subsequent study on 63 patients [31] indicated that only patients with epilepsy who also suffer from migraine and/or the hyperkinetic syndrome respond to dietary treatment, but not patients with epilepsy alone. It is possible that these patients suffer from an otherwise latent form of epilepsy which is activated by migraine-induced disturbances of cerebral perfusion. OLESEN et al. [54] and LAURITZEN et al. [45] observed cerebral hypoperfusion comparable to LEAOS', spreading depression in migraine. Similarly, focal cerebral hypoperfusion affecting mainly the frontal lobes was shown to occur in children with the hyperkinetic syndrome [48]. Although there was marked clinical improvement of the epilepsy and of migraine in these patients, there was little change on the EEG [31]. This and the fact that epilepsy did not improve as long as the patients continued to have headaches would support the hypothesis that migraine was the trigger of an otherwise latent epilepsy. Both epileptic seizures and migraine and/or hyperkinetic behaviour recurred reproducibly when provoking foods were eaten. In patients who responded to dietary treatment it was possible to phase out anticonvulsants without relapse of seizures. Although only the minority of epileptic patients who suffer from both epilepsy and migraine respond to dietary treatment, it is important because some may recover merely by avoiding certain foods.

Is it Allergy?

Most clinical immunologists prefer to restrict the term allergy to immunologically mediated intolerances, and some to IgE-mediated reactions only. Others, applying a more historical perspective [78], use it as a more general term for adverse reactions. Food allergy provoking symptoms of the CNS are not IgE-mediated, and no known immunological mechanisms have been identified to explain this association [29–31]. Moreover, the interval between eating a provoking food and appearance of symptoms may last several days, which from an immunological point of view is not easily explained. However, several features suggest allergy rather than other types of intolerance. (a) A wide variation of foods with, as far as we know, nothing in common can provoke symptoms. Indeed, the successful demonstration that these diseases are food-related, sprang from testing the deduction from the allergy hypothesis that any food in any combination can cause the symptoms. The combinations of foods observed suggested common antigenicity rather than common pharmacological effects. Children who reacted to cow's milk but not to goat's milk also reacted to cow's cheese but not to goat's cheese. (b) A food-allergy reaction can be "grown out of", which would not be expected from other types of intolerance. And (c) foods provoking symptoms of the CNS sometimes also provoke eczema, wheezing, and/or rhinitis.

In 1921 Prausnitz established by passive transfer of skin test response by serum that such food intolerance can be a food-allergic disease.

As the site of entry, one would expect the gastrointestinal tract to be especially prone to food-allergic disease. The absorption of intact antigen is a feature of normal gastrointestinal function. The amounts which enter the circulation are of no nutritional significance but are clearly sufficient to immunize, since antibodies to intact food proteins can be demonstrated in healthy individuals. It is assumed that the function of these antibodies is to eliminate safely those food antigens that do succeed in gaining access to the circulation. It is considered likely that the complexes formed by the combination of antibody and food antigen are removed from the blood by phagocytes, this sequence of events occuring asymptomatically after each meal. It seems possible that this system has broken down in the individual with food allergy, and symptoms may arise as a direct consequence of defective handling of normally harmless antigens which have entered the circulation by the gastrointestinal route [55].

However, allergy and idiosyncrasy may coexist, possibly one the effect of the other.

The Cytochrom P-450 Complex. Poor metabolizers have been seen in all populations, but there is considerable heterogeneity with respect to metabolic status. There is an increase in the frequency of slow metabolizers in Western populations and there is an increased incidence in food-allergic patients (BROSTOFF 1988, personal communication).

The Role of Food Phenolic Compounds. Cholerogenic acid (a phenol) which is found in green coffee, castor bean and oranges can produce an immediate wheal-and-flare reaction in sensitized subjects [37]. Phenolic compounds are in widespread use in may foods. LITTLEWOOD et al. [46] showed that the allele P of the phenolsulphotransferase in platelets is decreased during migraine attacks in patients with food-induced migraine. They speculated that increased amounts of phenolic compounds could accumulate if the gastrointestinal phenolsulphotransferase were similarly affected. Such a primary or acquired enzyme deficiency could alter antigen handling [1] or induce migraine directly.

Opioid Peptides. Although migraine has been viewed as a cerebrovascular disorder, there is growing evidence suggesting that the primary problem in migraine may be a selective change in brain metabolism [54]. What triggers the changes in neuronal metabolism is not known, but it is likely that peptidergic and opioid substances play a role [5, 32, 69]. Some of these neurotransmitters may derive from the gut or from foods; it was shown that brain levels of amino acid derived neurotransmitters can be affected by dietary precursors [85], and opiate-like peptides were discovered in a number of foods, especially in milk [8] and wheat [44]. Opioid peptides have also been implicated in the pathophysiology of epileptic seizures [38] and in the induction of mast cells [14, 67] – closing the circuit between food hypersensitivity, migraine and epilepsy.

The Role of Placebo. Diets may have a powerful placebo effect. Moreover, in humans and experimental animals allergic changes may become a conditioned reflex after repeated allergen exposure [27, 64]. These data suggest a two-way communication between mind and body, as well as between the CNS and the immune system [3]. However, the reproducible association of deterioration with certain foods is unlikely to be a placebo effect, nor are the results of the double-blind, placebo-controlled crossover trials.

Conclusion

Taken together, the available research suggests that particular types of adverse food reactions sometimes correlate with neurological and psychiatric symptoms. The diversity of foods involved, which apparently have nothing in common, is suggestive of allergy, and the adverse food effects may correlate with immunological abnormalities. However, diets may affect brain function in various ways.

Research into affective disorders has highlighted the importance of amino acid derived neurotransmitters in the regulation of brain function. It has shown that brain levels can be affected by dietary precursors [85]. On the other hand, it has been variously reported that these patients may suffer specific food cravings, addiction and withdrawal symptoms [60]. The discovery of opiate-like peptides in milk [8] and wheat [44] and a possible induction of mast cell degranulation by opiates [14] makes a relationship between food addiction and food allergy in some patients a possibility.

A similar relationship may exist between apparently food-allergic reactions and as yet poorly understood enzyme defects, such as that of the phenolsulphotransferase in platelets during food-induced migraine or the decreased activity of the cytochrom P-450 complex, which might lead to an abnormal metabolism of chemical compounds and other substances.

The Risks. Dietary management of the kind discussed is demanding and, if not properly supervised, dangerous due to malnutrition, anaphylaxis, status epilepticus, social disruption and the Münchhausen by proxy syndrome.

The Needs. Research needs include the further exploration of such management in other neurological and psychiatric disorders, avoiding the pitfall of the assumption that each syndrome must have a single cause. Research is needed to answer the question as to whether it is allergy or idiosyncrasy, or both, and to develop diagnostic tests and simpler methods of treatment.

References

1. Aalberse RC, Koshte V, Clements JGJ (1981) IgE antibodies that cross react with vegetable foods, pollens and hymenoptena venom. J Allergy Clin Immunol 68:356
2. Adamson WD, Sellers ED (1932) Observations on the incidence of a hypersensitive state in 100 cases of epilepsy. J Allergy 4:315–323
3. Ader R (1981) Psychoneuroimmunology. Academic, New York
4. American Psychiatric Association (1980) Diagnostic and statistical manual of mental disorders, 3rd edn. American Psychiatric Association, Washington DC, pp 42–44
5. Anthony M (1982) Serotonin and cyclic nucleotides in migraine. Adv Neurol 33:48
6. Bartrop RW, Luckhurst E, Lazarus L et al. (1977) Depressed lymphocyte function after bereavment. Lancet 1:834 836
7. Beauchemin JA (1935) Allergic reactions in mental diseases. Am J Psychiatry 92:1190
8. Brantl V, Teschenmacher HA (1979) A material with opioid activity in bovine milk and milk products. Naunyn Schmiedebergs Arch Phamacol 306:301–304
9. Brown RC (1920) The protein of foodstuffs as a factor in the cause of headache. Wis Med J 19:337
10. Campbell MB (1970) Allergy and epilepsy. In: Speer F (ed) Allergy of the nervous system. Thomas, Springfield IL, pp 59–78
11. Campbell MB (1973) Neurologic manifestations of allergic disease. Ann Allergy 31:485–498
12. Campbell MB (1974) Neurological and psychiatric aspects of allergy. Otolaryngol Clin North Am 7:805
13. Carter CM, Egger J, Soothill JF (1985) A dietary management of severe childhood migraine. Hum Nutr Appl Nutr 39 A:294–303
14. Casale TB, Bowmann S, Kaliner M (1984) Induction of human cutaneous mast cell degranulation by opiates and endogenous opioid peptides: evidence for opiate and non-opiate receptor participation. J Allergy Clin Immunol 73:775
15. Chobot R, Dundy HD, Pacella BL (1950) The incidence of abnormal electroencephalographic patterns in allergic children. J Allergy 21:334–338
16. Congdon PJ, Forsythe WI (1979) Migraine in childhood: a study of 300 children. Dev Med Child Neurjol 21:209–216
17. Conners CK (1973) Rating scales for use in drug studies with children. Psychopharmacol Bull 9:24–48
18. Conners CK, Goyette CH, Southwick DA et al. (1976) Food additives and hyperkinesis: a controlled double-blind experiment. Pediatrics 58:154–166
19. Cooke RA (1922) Studies in specific hypersensitiveness. On the phenomenon of hyposensitization (the clinically lessened sensitiveness of allergy). J Immunol 7:219
20. Crayton JW, Stone T, Stein G (1981) Epilepsy precipitated by food sensitivity: report of a case with double-blind placebocontrolled assessment. Clin Electroencephalogr 12:192–198
21. Crook WG, Harrison WW, Cawford SE, Emmerson BS (1961) Systemic manifestations due to allergy. Pediatrics 27:790–799
22. Cunningham AS (1975) Allergy, immunodeficiency and epilepsy. Lancet II:975

23. Davison HM (1952) Allergy of the nervous system. Q Rev Allergy Immunol 6:157–188
24. Dees SC (1953) Electroencephalography in jallergic epilepsy. South Med J 46:618-620
25. Dees SC (1954) Neurologic allergy in childhood. Pediatr Clin North Am 1:1017–1027
26. Dees SC, Loewenbach H (1951) Allergic epilepsy. Ann Allergy 9:446–458
27. Dekker E, Pelser HE, Grosen J (1957) Conditioning as a cause of asthmatic attacks: a laboratory study. J Psychosom Res 2:97–108
28. Dohan FC, Grasberger JC (1973) Relapsed schizophrenics: earlier discharge from the hospital after cereal-free milk-free diet. Am J Psychiatry 130:685–688
29. Egger J, Carter CM, Wilson J et al. (1983) Is migraine food allergy? A double-blind controlled trial of oligoantigenic diet treatment. Lancet II:868–869
30. Egger J, Carter CM, Graham PJ, Gamley D, Soothill JF (1985) Controlled trial of oloigoantigenic diet treatment in the hyperkinetic syndrome. Lancet 1:540–545
31. Egger J, Carter CM, Soothill JF, Wilson J (1988) Oligoantigenic diet treatment in children with epilepsy and migraine. J Pediatr (in press)
32. Fanchamps A (1982) The evolution of thinking about the role and site of action of serotonin in migraine. Adv Neurol 33:31–33
33. Fein BT, Kamin PB (1968) Allergy, convulsive disorders, and epilepsy. Ann Allergy 26:241–247
34. Feingold BF (1975) Hyperkinesis and learning disabilities linked to artificial food flavours and colors. Am J Nurs 75:797–803
35. Flintoff MM, Barron Rw, Swanson JM et al. (1982) Methylphenidate increases selectivity of visual scanning in children referred for hyperactivity. J Abnorm Child Psychol 10:145–163
36. Fowler WM, Heimlich EM, Walter RD et al. (1962) Electroencephalographic patterns in children with allergic convulsive and behaviour disorders. Ann Allergy 20:1–14
37. Freedman SO, Siddiavi JH, Krupey JH, Sehon AH (1962) Identification of a simple chemical compound (chlorogenic acid) as an allergen in plant material causing human atopic disease. Am J Med Sci 244:548
38. Frank H, Engel J, Ackerman RF, Shavit Y, Liebeskind JC (1979) Endogenous opioids may mediate post-ictal behavioural depression in amygdaloid kindlet rats. Brain Res 167:435–440
39. Grant HEC (1977) Food allergies and migraine. Lancet I:966–969
40. Hafer H (1984) Nahrungsphosphat - Die heimliche Droge. Ursache für Verhaltensstörungen, Schulversagen und Jugendkriminalität. Kriminalistik, Heidelberg
41. Hannington E (1967) Preliminary report on tyramine headache. Br Med J II:550–551
42. Harley PJ, Ray RS, Tomasi L et al. (1978) Hypokinesis and food additives: testing the Feingold hypothesis. Pediatrics 61:818–828
43. Hoobler BR (1916) Some early symptoms suggesting protein sensitization in infancy. Am J Dis Child (1979) 12:129
44. Klee WA, Zioudrou, Streaty RA (1979) Exorphins: peptides with opioid activity isolated from wheat gluten, and their possible role in the etiology of schizophrenia. In: Usdin E, Bunney WE, Kline NS (eds) Endophins in mental health research. Oxford University Press, New York, pp 209–218
45. Lauritzen M, Olesen J (1984) Regional cerebral blood flow during migraine attacks by xenon-133 inhalation and emission tomography. Brain 107:447–461

46. Littlewood J, Glover V, Sandler M (1982) Platelet phenolsulfotransferase deficiency in dietary migraine. Lancet I:983–986
47. Liveing E (1873) On megrim, sick headaches and some allied disorders. Churchill, London
48. Lou HC, Henriksen L, Bruhn P (1984) Focal cerebral hypoperfusion in children with dysphasia and/or attention deficit disorder. Arch Neurol 41:825–828
49. Macharness R (1976) Not all in the mind. Pan Books, London
50. Mendelson W, Johnson N, Stewart M (1971) Hyperactive children as teenagers: a follow up study. J Nerv Ment Dis 153:237–239
51. Menkes MM, Rowe JS, Menkes JH (1967) A twenty-five year follow-up study on the hyperkinetic child with minimal brain dysfunction. Pediatrics 39:393–399
52. Minot GR (1923) The role of low carbohydrate diet in the treatment of migraine and headache. Med Clin North Am 7:715
53. Monro J, Brostoff J, Carini C, Zilkha KJ (1980) Food allergy in migraine. Lancet II:1–4
54. Olesen J, Larsen B, Lauritzen M (1981) Focal hyperemia followed by spreading oligemia and impaired activation of rCBF in classic migraine. Ann Neurol 9:344–352
55. Paganelli R, Levinsky RJ, Atherton DJ (1981) Detection of specific antigen within circulating immune complexes. Validation of the assay and its application to food antigen-antibody complexes found in healthy and food allergic subjects. Clin Exp Immunol 46:44–53
56. Pagniez P, Vallery-Raddt P, Nast A (1919) Therapeutique preventative de certaines migraine. Presse Med 27:172
57. Potkin SG, Weinberger D, Kleinman J et al. (1981) Wheat-gluten challenge in schizophrenic patients. Am J Psychatry 138:1208–1211
58. Prior M, Griffin M (1985) Hyperactivity. Diagnosis and management. Heinemann Medical, London
59. Randolph TG (1947) Allergy as a causative factor for fatigue, irritability, and behaviour problems of children. J Pediatr 31:560–572
60. Randolph TG (1978) Specific adaptation. Ann Allergy 40:333–345
61. Rapp DJ (1979) Allergies and the hyperactive child. Simon and Shuster, New York
62. Rowe AH (1931) Food allergy, its manifestations, diagnosis and treatment. Lea and Febinger, Philadelphia
63. Rowe AH (1950) Allergic toxemia and fatigue. Ann Allergy 8:22
64. Russel M, Dark KA, Cummins RW et al. (1984) Learned histamine release. Science 225:733–734
65. Sandler MMBH, Hannington E (1974) A phenyl-aethylamine oxidising defect in migraine. Nature 250:335–337
66. Schoenthaler SJ (1983) Diet and delinquency: a multi-staste replication. Int J Biosoc Res 5:70–117
67. Shanahan F, Lee TDG, Binenstock J, Befus AD (1984) The influence of endorphins on peritoneal and mucosal cell secretion. J Allergy Clin Immunol 74:499
68. Sheldon JM, Randolph TG (1935) Allergy in migraine-like headaches. Am J Med Sci 190–232
69. Sicuteri F (1982) Natural opioids in migraine. Adv Neurol 33
70. Spangler RH (1927) Allergy and epilepsy. J Lab Clin Med 12:41–58
71. Speer F (1970) Allergy of the nervous system. Thomas, Springfield IL

72. Sternberg TH, Baldridge GD (1948) Electroencephalograpic abnormalities in patients with generalized neurodermatitis. J Invest Dermatol 11:401-403
73. Swanson JM, Kinsbourne M (1980) Food dyes impair performance of hyperactive children on a laboratory learning test. Science 207:1485-1487
74. Terrel CO, Stephens WE, Morris R (1967) Eosinophilia and neurological dysfunction - a preliminary report. Ann Allergy 25:673-677
75. Thompson J (1921) Clinical types of convulsive seizures in very young babies with a special consideration of so-called idiopathic convulsions of early infancy and their treatment. Br Med J II:679-683
76. Thorley G (1984) Pilot study to assess behavioural and cognitive effects of artificial food colours in a group of retarded children. Dev Med Child Neurol (1952) 26:56-61
77. Unger AH, Unger L (1952) Migraine is an allergic disease. J Allergy 23:429-440
78. van Pirquet CE (1906) Allergie. Klin Wochenschr 53:1457
79. Wallis RM, Nicol WD, Craig M (1923) The importance of protein hypersensitivity in the diagnosis and treatment of a special group of epileptics. Lancet I:741-743
80. Walther B (1984) Nahrungsphosphat und Verhaltensstörung im Kindesalter. Ergebnisse einer kontrollierten Diätstudie. In: Steinhausen HC (ed) Das konzentrationsgestörte und hyperaktive Kind. Kohlhammer, Stuttgart
81. Ward JF, Peterson HA (1927) Protein sensitization in epilepsy. Arch Neurol Psychiatry 17:427-443
82. Weiss B, Williams JH, Margen S et al. (1980) Behavioral response to artificial food colors. Science 207:1487-1489
83. Weiss G, Minde K, Werry JS et al. (1971) Studies on the hyperactive child. VIII. 5 year follow-up. Arch Gen Psychiatry 24:409-414
84. Williams JJ, Cram DM, Tausig FT, Webster E (1978) Relative affects of drugs and diet on hyperactive behaviors: an experimental study. Pediatrics 61:811-817
85. Wurtmann RJ (1983) Behavioural effects of nutrients. Lancet 1:1145-1147

The Relevance of History for the Diagnosis of Cow's Milk Allergy: A Prospective Study in Danish Infants

A. Høst

Previous studies on the incidence of cow's milk allergy (CMA) have produced considerably varying figures, ranging from about 0.5% to 7.5%. Many of the studies were not carried out prospectively; an example is the study by Stintzing and Zetterström [1], who reported an incidence of CMA of 0.5%. In other studies the diagnosis of CMA has been based mainly on patient history, for example, that by Gerrard et al. [2], giving an incidence of CMA of 7.5%. In a prospective study, Jacobsson and Lindberg [3] determined the incidence of CMA to be 1.9%, based on the results of well-defined elimination/challenge procedures.

The aims of the present study were (a) to investigate the incidence of CMA in infants in an urban Danish community, (b) to record in detail the type of early feeding, and (c) to examine the relevance of clinical history for the diagnosis of CMA based on strict elimination/challenge procedures. CMA, as used here, refers to reproducible adverse reactions to cow's milk (CM), whether of IgE-mediated or non-IgE-mediated type; the diagnosis of CMA was based on the results of elimination and open challenge studies following generally accepted criteria [4, 5].

Patients and Methods

Odense, a city on the island of Fünen in Denmark, has about 173000 inhabitants. Some 1800 infants are born there each year. It has one obstetric and one children's hospital. All infants born during 1985 to mothers living in the municipality of Odense at the time of birth were followed during the 1st year of life. A total of 1758 infants were born alive (99.2% at the University Hospital), and 9 died neonatally; 1749 were followed up. Before the beginning of the study, all general practitioners and practising paediatricians in Odense were informed of the investigation by letter, and all 20 health visitors were thoroughly informed by meetings and in writing, and all agreed to participate.

At the hospital the mothers of all 1749 newborns received both oral and written information about the study. The mothers were asked to contact their health visitor in case of one or more of the following symptoms in the infants: recurrent wheezing, rhinitis, exzema, urticaria, erythema/exanthema, vomiting and/or diarrhoea not due to coincidental infection or other demonstrable cause, infantile colic not disappearing after advice on feeding technique, and failure to thrive. If the suspicion of CMA was confirmed by the health visitor and the family doctor, the infants were referred to the Paediatric Clinic of the University Hospital. During the study period, more than 99% of the infants were followed regularly during the 1st year of life by health visitors. One infant died, and 14 left the municipality, none of whom developed symptoms of CMA.

Clinical Examinations. At referral all infants were examined by the same doctor. The following data were obtained: family history of atopy and a case history, including a careful dietary history with special regard to type of early feeding and introduction of CM products. Further, records from the newborn nursery were reviewed for dietary history.

Laboratory Analyses. Cord blood IgE (Phadebas IgE, Prist) was determined routinely during 1985. Moreover, the analyses were performed: haemoglobin, IgE, specific IgE against CM (radioallergosorbent test, Al-RAST), skin prick test, and β-lactoglobulin in human milk (enzyme-linked immunosorbent assay, ELISA).

Diagnostic Criteria. The diagnosis of CMA was established according to the following criteria: (a) definite disappearance of symptoms after each of two dietary eliminations of CM, (b) recurrence of identical symptoms after one challenge, and (c) exclusion of lactose intolerance and coincidental infection. A milk-free diet was maintained for at least 4 weeks before milk challenge. All challenges were initiated in the hospital under professional observation. The challenge procedure was open. In exclusively breast-fed infants elimination/challenge was performed via the mother's intake of CM. In formula-fed infants the challenge was with Allomin (a CM-based formula 15 g/l; casein/whey, 4/6) in the following dosage: at 0 h, 5 ml; at 2 h, 10 ml; at 4 h, 20 ml; at 6 h, 40 ml; and at 8 h, 80 ml. If no symptoms had occurred after 8 h (and after a total dose of 155 ml Allomin), the child was sent home, with increasing amounts (80–160 ml) to be taken at home until customary daily intake of milk product was tolerated. If late reactions occurred at home, the patient was reinvestigated in hospital as soon as possible, and at a suspected reaction to CM the last dose was repeated once. During elimination of CM a casein hydrolysate (Nutramigen) was used as a milk substitute, unless the infant could be fully breast fed.

Once the diagnosis of CMA had been confirmed a milk-free diet was continued until a new milk challenge was performed at the age of 12 months. It was also recommended to avoid introduction of solid foods until the age of 6 months and highly allergenic foods as fish, citrus, eggs, tomatoes, strawberries, chocolate, nuts, berries, peas and beans until the age of 12 months.

Results

The results of elimination/challenge procedures in 117 admitted infants (6.7% of all followed up) with symptoms suggestive of CMA showed that 39 had reproducible adverse reactions to CM, giving an incidence of CMA of 2.2% (39/1749) in the 1st year of life. Of these 39 infants, 17 developed symptoms of CMA during breast feeding, in all cases before the age of 3 months. Nine of these were solely breast fed at the time of diagnosis, giving a 1-year incidence of CMA in exclusively breast-fed infants of 0.5% (9/1749) in a study population with a frequency of exclusive breast feeding of 52% at 3 months age. In 67% (78/117) the suspicion of CMA was not confirmed; one had lactose intolerance; 12 did not improve on milk-free diet. A total of 65 who apparently became symptomfree on a milk-free diet remained symptom free after challenge.

Comparing the group of infants with confirmed CMA to the group consisting of infants with non-confirmed CMA, the former was characterized by infants with an earlier onset of symptoms (median, 1 month versus 3 months; range, 1 week to 8 months versus 1 week to 12 months) and a higher frequency of positive skin prick test against CM (41% versus 3%). No differences were found concerning sex, elevation of cord blood IgE, atopic predisposition or specific IgE to CM (Table 1). Data on early feeding (Table 2) do not differ regarding the percentages of infants never breast fed or exclusively breast fed at 3 months of age. However, *all infants* with confirmed CMA had received occasional supplements of CM formula during the first 3 days of life (median, 185 ml Allomin; range, 40–860 ml), while "only" 87% of the

Table 1. Clinical data on 117 infants with symptoms suggestive of CMA

	Infants with confirmed CMA ($n=39$)	Infants with non-confirmed CMA ($n=78$)
Sex	20 girls/19 boys	40 girls/38 boys
Cord blood IgE $\geqslant$0.5 ku/l	8 (21%)	18 (23%)
Atopic predisposition	18 (46%)	28 (36%)
Positive skin prick test to cow's milk[a]	16 (41%)	2 (3%)
Specific IgE to cow's milk (Al-RAST $\geqslant$ 2)	12 (31%)	20 (26%)
Age at onset of symptoms		
Median	1 month	3 months
Range	1 week to 8 months	1 week to 12 months

[a] $p < .05$ (χ^2 test)

Table 2. Early feeding in 117 infants with symptoms suggestive of CMA

	Infants with confirmed CMA ($n=39$)	Infants with non-confirmed CMA ($n=78$)
Never breast fed	7 (18%)	14 (18%)
Exclusively breast fed at 3 months	17 (44%)	36 (46%)
Supplements of cow's milk formula neonatally	39 (100%)	68 (87%)

infants with non-confirmed CMA had ingested supplements of CM formula neonatally in the newborn nursery.

Cutaneous symptoms were the most common (64%) among infants with confirmed CMA (Table 3), followed by gastrointestinal reactions (59%) and respiratory reactions (33%). In infants with non-confirmed CMA 49% had cutaneous, 37% gastrointestinal and only 22% respiratory symptoms. The most striking difference between the two groups was the occurrence of monosymptomatology in only 3 infants (8%) with confirmed CMA versus 46 (59%) among infants with non-confirmed CMA.

At the age of 12 months, 22 (56%) of the 39 infants with confirmed CMA did not react at milk challenge, and at 18 months a further 6 (a total of 72%) tolerated CM.

In the overall study population (1749 infants) the frequency of exclu-

Table 3. Symptomatology in 117 infants with symptoms suggestive of CMA

	Infants with confirmed CMA ($n=39$)	Infants with non-confirmed CMA ($n=78$)
Cutaneous symptoms		
Total	25 (64%)	38 (49%)
Eczema	22 (56%)	36 (46%)
Urticaria	6 (15%)	4 (5%)
Eczema and urticaria	4 (10%)	2 (3%)
Respiratory symptoms		
Total	13 (33%)	17 (22%)
Recurrent wheezing	11 (28%)	15 (19%)
Rhinitis	8 (21%)	11 (14%)
Recurrent wheezing and rhinitis[a]	6 (15%)	2 (3%)
Gastrointestinal symptoms		
Total	23 (59%)	29 (37%)
Infantile colic	18 (46%)	17 (22%)
Vomitus[a]	15 (38%)	12 (15%)
Diarrhoea	3 (8%)	7 (9%)
Monosymptomatology[a]	3 (8%)	46 (59%)

[a] $p<.05$ (χ^2 test)

sive breast feeding was as follows: 70% at 1 month, 61% at 2 months, 52% at 3 months, 49% at 4 months, 29% at 5 months and 21% at 6 months. However, review of records from the newborn nursery revealed that 1539 (88%) newborns had ingested varying amounts of CM formula during the first 3 days of life, and that all 39 infants with confirmed CMA had ingested CM formula neonatally. All nine infants with CMA against CM protein in human milk had received "inadvertent" supplements of CM formula during their stay in the newborn nursery in spite of sufficient breast milk. None of the 210 neonates without supplements of CM formula developed CMA.

Discussion

In this study the 1-year incidence of CMA in infants was 2.2%, and the incidence of CMA in exclusively breast-fed infants was 0.5%. Both figures are comparable with the corresponding figures in the study of JACOBSSON and LINDBERG [3], who reported the total incidence of CMA to be 1.9% and the incidence of CMA in exclusively breast-fed infants to be 0.4% (45% entirely breast fed at 3 months of age).

In 117 infants with symptoms suggestive of CMA the suspicion could be disproven in 78 (67%) by a practical approach including elimination and open milk challenge procedures. Recently, Bock [6] has reported similar findings in a prospective study of the natural history of adverse reactions to foods among 480 children during the first 3 years of life. In his study, 72 (15%) had adverse reactions suggestive of CMA, and 25 (5.2%) had reproducible reactions on challenge with CM – 11 confirmed by blind challenge (2.2%) and 14 (3%) confirmed by open challenge. Reproducible reactions on open milk challenge were not observed in 47 (65%).

It is noteworthy that all 39 infants with confirmed CMA in our study had ingested CM formula during the first 3 days of life. The nine infants with CMA against CM protein in human milk (all exclusively breast fed at the time of discharge from the newborn nursery and at the time of diagnosis) had been exposed neonatally to CM formula in amounts corresponding to approximately 0.4–3.0 g β-lactoglobulin. Using ELISA, detectable amounts (0.5–45 ng/ml) were found in 3/9 samples of human milk against which the infants reacted clinically. Early inadvertent and occasional exposure to CM proteins may possibly initiate sensitization in predisposed neonates. Subsequent exposure to minute amounts of CM proteins in human milk may act as booster doses eliciting allergic reactions.

Summary and Conclusion

A cohort of 1749 newborns in the municipality of Odense were followed prospectively for the development of CMA during their 1st year of life. In all, 39 (2.2%) fulfilled the criteria for CMA based on the results of elimination and open milk challenge procedures, whereas 78 (67%) of 117 infants with symptoms suggestive of CMA did not show reproducible symptoms on elimination and open milk challenge procedures.

Of the 39 infants with confirmed CMA, nine were solely breast fed at the time of diagnosis, giving a 1-year incidence of CMA in exclusively breast-fed infants of 0.5% (9/1749) in a study population with a frequency of exclusive breast feeding of 52% at 3 months of age.

None of the infants had signs of CMA during the 1st week of life. In comparison with the group of 78 infants without reproducible symptoms of CMA, the 39 infants with confirmed CMA were characterized by a significantly higher frequency of positive skin prick test to CM protein, an earlier onset of symptoms, (median, 1 month), a significantly higher frequency of recurrent wheezing combined with rhinitis, a significantly higher frequency of vomitus, and the presence of two or more symptoms suggestive of CMA.

Of the 1749 infants, 1539 (88%) had ingested varying amounts of CM formula during the first 3 days of life, often in spite of sufficient nursing. All 39 infants with confirmed CMA had received CM formula (at least partly), even if most of the infants were breast fed at discharge from the nursery. Early occasional exposure to CM proteins may possibly initiate sensitization in predisposed neonates.

References

1. Stintzing G, Zetterström R (1979) Cow's milk allergy, incidence and pathogenetic role of early exposure to cow's milk formula. Acta Paediatr Scand 68:383–387
2. Gerrard JW, MacKenzie JWA, Goluboff N (1973) Cow's milk allergy: prevalence and manifestations in an unselected series of newborns. Acta Paediatr Scand (Suppl) 234:3–21
3. Jacobsson I, Lindberg T (1979) A prospective study of cow's milk protein intolerance in Swedish infants. Acta Paediatr Scand 68:853–859.
4. Bahna SL, Gandhi MD (1983) Milk hypersensitivity. II. Practical aspects of diagnosis, treatment and prevention. Ann Allergy 50:295–301
5. Savilahti E (1981) Cow's milk allergy. Allergy 36:73–88.
6. Bock SA (1987) Prospective appraisal of complaints of adverse reactions to foods in children during the first 3 years of life. Pediatrics 79:683–688.

References

IgE-Mediated Allergies

R. Urbanek

Introduction

IgE-mediated immune reactions are but one kind of allergic reaction. In this early-reaction type the IgE, which is bound to the surface of mast cells and basophil granulocytes, is responsible both for allergen-antibody induced degranulation and for the release of mediators. Medical symptoms depend, on the one hand, on the degree of the patient's sensitivity and, on the other, on the respective manner in which the allergen enters the body. IgE-mediated reactions cause the development of obstructive bronchitis and rhinoconjunctivitis in the respiratory tract and can cause vomiting, diarrhea, and severe colic in the gastrointestinal tract.

Abnormal reactions to foodstuffs are identifiable by pathological responses to ingested food or food additives. *Food allergy* is an immunologicaly mediated response which has no relationship to the physiological reaction resulting from ingested foods. To date, study of IgE-mediated reactions has served as the only practical means of sufficiently understanding immunological mechanisms. *Nutritional intolerance* is not an immunologically mediated response; it can result either from a pharmacologic or metabolic mechanisms or from contamination with microorganisms (Table 1).

Table 1. Classification of abnormal responses to food

Intolerance
Intoxication
Celiac disease
Lactase deficiency
Allergy
Delayed type reaction
Immediate type reaction

IgE-mediated reactions to nutritional allergens are found principally during the first years of life in infants affected by atopy. In industrialized countries the number of children suffering from food allergies is estimated to average 5% (0.3%–7.5%) [1, 3, 4], range higher in the case of atopy sufferers than in that of nonsufferers. About 10% of the atopic population develop clinical food allergy symptoms; in the case of atopic dermatitis or children with bronchial asthma the incidence is 25% [7]. However, asymptomatic sensitivity, in which no symptoms arise during the exercise tolerance test, must be distinguished from the symptomatic form. Among those foodstuffs which provoke an immediate allergic reaction during infancy, special attention should be given to egg and cow's milk. Both of these foodstuffs are frequently found as an ingredient in other foods. Accordingly, sensitivity to these proteins may arouse symptoms in the gastrointestinal tract as well as in other organs.

Immunological Response to Food Allergens

Every day large quantities of nutritional allergens are processed by the gastrointestinal tract. With the aid of digestive enzymes the proteins are reduced to molecules which no longer have immunogenicity. The absorption of nondegraded proteins by the intestines is prevented by the local defense mechanisms and the secretory IgA. Because the intestinal defense is incomplete, nutritional antigens can enter the body of healthy as well as susceptible persons and result in an immunological response triggered by the formation of antibodies. The highest level of antibodies to nutritional proteins is observed among children whose intestinal defenses show either functional or anatomic disorders. In addition to atopy-affected patients, sufferers with celiac disease, Crohn's disease, and children with long-lasting infectious gastroenteritis are also affected.

Specific IgE antibodies are usually not found; these are, however, being found increasingly in atopy-affected patients. Furthermore, most patients with atopic dermatitis are susceptible to an associated sensitivity to nutritional as well as inhalable allergens. However, this sensitivity must be examined individually to determine its clinical relevance. Specific IgE antibodies to egg albumin proteins as well as to components such as ovalbumin and ovomucoid are considered unfavorable indicators in the prognosis of long-term atopic dermatitis.

Specific IgA and IgG antibodies are the result of oral antigen intake by individuals and those with damaged gastrointestinal mucosa. When an active immunological condition has been attained, the immunological response to renewed exposure to the gastrointestinal antigen may occur, although this may or may not disturb either the anatomic structure or the functioning of the gastrointestinal tract. This consequently leads to the conclusion, that a specific immunological response to oral antigens/allergens may only be regarded as pathological if found in combination with anatomic and functional mucous damage [2, 6].

Medical Symptoms

Allergic symptoms may appear after a few minutes (early-reaction type), after hours (delayed-reaction type), or after a few days (late-reaction type). The most common cutaneous are itching, erythema, paleness, urticarial eruptions, and local swelling. Gastrointestinal symptoms include colic, nausea, vomiting, and diarrhea. In the respiratory tract rhinoconjunctivitis, laryngitis, and bronchial illnesses such as coughing and angina pectoris may occur. Children seldom have systematic cardiovascular reactions, although the symptoms described may occur at any age. The most common pathologic allergy symptoms during childhood are mucocutaneous symptoms, rhinitis, and obstructive bronchitis. Increased levels of specific IgE are generally found in the so-called early-reaction type of responses. Symptoms exclusive to gastrointestinal illnesses, especially those of the delayed-reaction type, are seldom accompanied by IgE-mediated sensitivity.

Diagnostic Methods

In most cases diagnosis is based on the current symptoms and the anamnesis. Diagnostic in vivo and in vitro methods are employed to help identify the pathogenic nutrient (Table 2).

Food-specific IgE antibodies and other IgE antibodies may be identified through radioimmunoassay (RIA), enzyme immunoassay (EIA), or fluorescence immunoassay. During childhood the status of serum antibodies provides only nominal diagnostic assistance. The medical relevance of immunological findings must always be examined in relationship to the patient's medical history and the results of challenge tests. Not only cow's milk but also soya milk can induce the formation of specific antibodies in infants. According to May et al. [5], no preventive effect against the formation of cow's milk specific antibodies could be obtained when infants, who were initially breast fed or fed soya milk, were later given cow's milk.

Specific IgG antibodies to foodstuffs are found in healthy as well as in atopy-affected persons. An increased occurence of IgG antibodies to foodstuffs was observed with atopic dermatitis. It has been questioned whether an increased intestinal permeability is responsible for the formation of specific IgG antibodies to nutritive proteins, but, in contrast, the gastrointestinal symptoms are not increased in patients with eczema.

IgG antibodies which result from nutritive allergens do not always belong to all IgG subclasses; the highest level of antibodies is found in the IgG1 and IgG4 subclasses. Interestingly, lower levels of IgG4 to cow's milk are found in infants who have an early-reaction type of allergy and IgE sensitivity. It must be reiterated that, in addition to the atopic disposition and the individual immunological response, the increased permeability and antigenic properties of the introduced allergens themselves exert an influence on the level of specific IgG and IgG-subclass antibodies.

Conclusions

In addition to the amount of allergen introduced, the immunological response is also influenced by the manner in which the allergen enters the human body. The processing of the antigen in the intestines, which is similar to the transformations resulting from cooking, baking, or hydrolysis, reduces the immunological response to the antigen concerned. The individual immune response is also responsible for the formation of excessive antibodies. For this reason it is necessasry that we critically interpret the immunological results obtained. Furthermore, it is not the sensitivity but the specification which poses the main problem when

Table 2. Diagnostic procedures in the case of abnormal responses to food

In vivo	Oral provocation skin test	Small-intestinal biopsy (with and without gliadin consumption)
In vitro	Specific IgE, IgG antibodies	Specific IgA, IgG antibodies
Positive in	Allergy	Celiac disease

interpreting the results of diverse methods of immunological research. Antibody-mediated as well as nonimmunological mechanisms can lead to allergic reactions and intolerance symptoms to nutritive or inhalable allergens.

References

1. Bahna SL, Heiner DC (1980) Allergies to milk. Grune & Stratton, New York, 1-3
2. Bürgin-Wolf A, Singer E, Friess HM, Berger R, Birbaumer A, Just M (1980) The diagnostic significance of antibodies to various cow's milk proteins. Eur J Pediatr 133:17-24
3. Gerrard JW, Mackenzie JWA, Goluboff N (1973) Cow's milk allergy: prevalence and manifestation in an unselected series of newborns. Acta Paediatr Scand [Suppl] 234:1-21
4. Goldman AS, Anderson DW Jr, Sellars WA, Saperstein S, Kniker WI, Halpern SR (1983) Milk allergy. I. Oral challenge with milk and isolated milk proteins in allergic children. Pediatrics 32:425-443
5. May CD, Fomon SJ, Remigio L (1982) Immunologic consequences of feeding infants with cow milk and soy products. Acta Paediatr Scand 72:43-71
6. Urbanek R (1986) Diagnostisches Vorgehen bei abnormen Reaktionen auf Nahrungsmittel und Nahrungsmittelzusätze. Monatsschr Kinderheilkd 134:779-786
7. Zeiger RS (1981) Atopic dermatitis of childhood: current concepts and management. Immunol Allergy Pract 3:39-51

Relationship of Histamine Release and Other In Vitro Methods to Oral Provocation Test in Hen's Egg Allergic Patients

S. Lau and U. Wahn

The diagnosis of food allergy is difficult because of the complex composition of foods and the lack of standardized extracts for testing as well as the variety of symptoms which are hard to reproduce. Only about one-third of suspected adverse reactions to food are actually allergic, i.e. IgE-mediated [2]. A large percentage of patients with specific IgE and positive skin test do not show any symptoms upon food challenge [16].

Hypersensitivity reactions to cow's milk and hen's egg represent the clinically most important food allergies during early childhood [7, 15, 16]. Most children sensitive to hen's egg are allergic to egg white, which contains most of the major allergens [1, 9, 11] (Table 1). Ovalbumin, ovomucoid (a trypsin inhibitor), ovotransferrin (conalbumin) and lysozyme have been identified by Langeland [11–13], Hofman [9] and Anet [1] as major allergens, representing approximately 80% of total protein. Their biochemical properties are well known. These four allergens can be found in raw and boiled egg [9]. Ovalbumin is the strongest allergen and available in a highly purified form and is, therefore, very suitable for controlled studies.

Using ovalbumin as a model, we studied the diagnostic value of in vitro methods for predicting the clinical relevance of a sensitization to hen's egg by comparing the outcome of a titrated oral provocation test to ovalbumin with serum concentrations of IgE, IgG1, and IgG4 anti-

Table 1. Allergenic proteins in hen's egg white

	% Protein	Molecular weight
Ovalbumin	65	36000
Ovomucoid	4	27000
Ovotransferrin	?	78000
Lysozyme	11	21000

bodies to ovalbumin as well as with histamine release data from mixed leukocytes. The histamine release method has been described as a rather sensitive technique to determine basophil sensitivity and the potency of an allergenic extract [14].

Material and Methods

We investigated 27 children; their ages ranged from 3.5 months to 12 years, and the ratio of boys to girls was 18:9. They were tested with serum IgE antibodies to hen's egg white (radioallergosorbent test, RAST, ≥ 2). All children had a positive history of egg allergy. Of the 27 children, 22 had atopic eczema, two bronchial asthma, two atopic eczema and asthma, and one presented with acute urticaria. Specific IgE and IgG subclass antibodies were measured by an enzyme-linked immunosorbent assay by Dr. URBANEK, Freiburg [10]. Titrated oral porovocation test was performed when the patient's clinical condition had stabilized. Egg had been excluded from the died for at least 1 week prior to the provocation procedure. Lyophilized ovalbumin was portioned and stored in opaque capsules. For provocation, ovalbumin was dissolved in approximately 5 ml tea. An initial dose of 1 mg ovalbumin was used. If no response occurred within 30 min, the ten-fold dose was given, up to a maximum of 1 g ovalbumin. The patients had to stay in hospital for at least 24 h after provocation to document possible late reactions.

After dextran sedimentation of patient's blood, the upper layer containing leukocytes, platelets and plasma was washed in buffer, and the cells were incubated with serial dilutions of ovalbumin at concentrations ranging from 0.0001 to 10 µg/ml (ovalbumin was from Sigma, Munich in its purest available form). The tubes were incubated in 37 °C bath. After 40 min incubation the tubes were centrifuged and the supernatants decanted and assayed for histamine. Histamine was assayed by an automated fluorometric technique as described by SIRAGANIAN [17]. Basophil sensitivity – Ag_{30}, i.e. the antigen concentration necessary to release 30% of cellular histamine – was determined.

Results

During provocation procedure only immediate reactions were noticed, i.e. those occurring between 2 and 20 min after challenge. None of the children showed a late reaction. Of the 27 children, 17 responded to the ovalbumin challenge (six at 10 mg, five at 100 mg, and six at 1 g). Ten children showed no response. Twelve of the children with a positive challenge test showed a significant (>30%) histamine release from leukocytes while five of this group were negative up to an allergen concentration of 10 μg/ml. Six of the ten children with a negative oral provocation test released histamine from basophils, and four did not. Figure 1 shows the positive histamine release of a patient with positive oral provocation.

There was no significant difference in the median value for Ag_{30} of children with positive oral provocation test and children with negative oral provocation test (Fig. 2). No correlation could be found between the threshold concentration of ovalbumin required for a positive oral provocation test and for a positive histamine release to ovalbumin.

The values for ovalbumin specific IgE, IgG1, and IgG4 antibodies covered a wide range. The mean values for ovalbumin specific serum IgE, IgG1 and IgG4, IgG1/IgG4 ratio and IgE/IgG4 ratio were higher

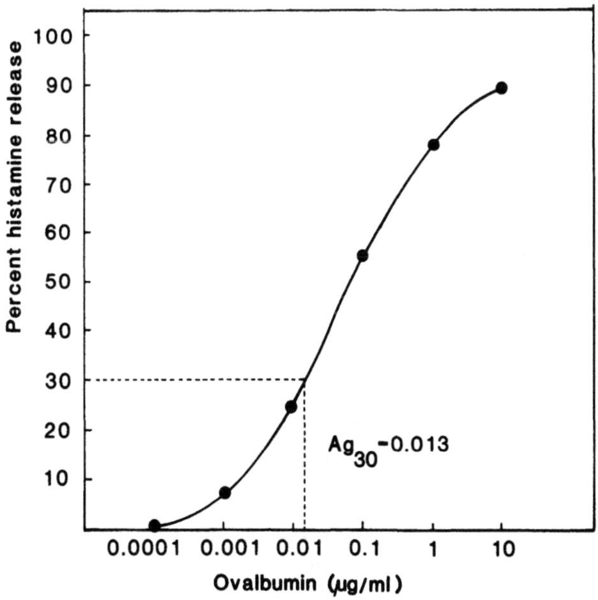

Fig. 1. Ovalbumin-induced histamine release from washed leukocytes of a hen's egg allergic patient. The patient was 36 months old and had atopic dermatitis. Serum IgE to hen's egg, RAST class 3; specific serum IgE to ovalbumin >50 AU; oral provocation with 1 g ovalbumin produced urticaria

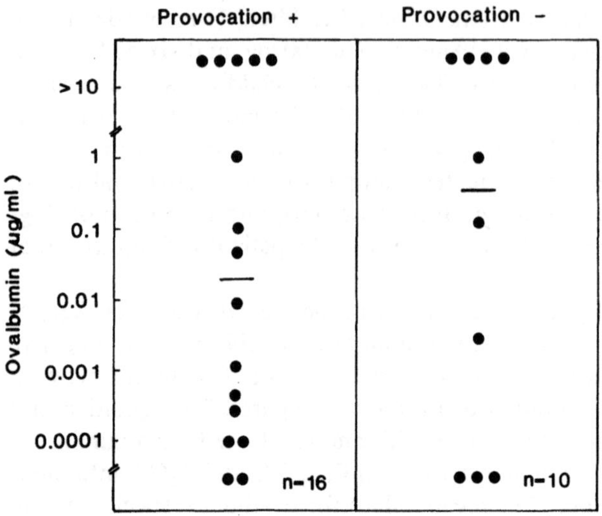

Fig. 2. Basophil sensitivity, expressed as the ovalbumin concentration necessary for 30 percent histamine release (Ag_{30}) in two groups of children, with positive and negative provocation test

in those children with a positive challenge test, but only the difference in the IgE/IgG4 ratio was statistically significant ($p<0.025$). Children with positive oral provocation test tended to be younger (not significant; Table 2). There was a positive correlation between the results of ovalbumin-induced histamine release and levels of specific serum IgE ($r=0.7$).

Table 2. Age and immunological data of children with positive and negative oral provocation test to ovalbumin

Mean values	Positive oral provocation ($n=17$)	Negative oral provocation ($n=10$)
Age (months)	24.4 ± 26.5	45.9 ± 48.8
Basophil sensitivity	0.1 ± 0.3 ($n=11$)	0.19 ± 0.4 ($n=6$)
Specific IgE (AU)	27.5 ± 22.0	17.0 ± 15.4
Specific IgG1 (AU)	1428.4 ± 2152.97	990.3 ± 1092.84
Specific IgG4 (AU)	417.4 ± 621.79	668.0 ± 1143.6
IgG1/IgG4 ratio	12.98 ± 25.77	7.2 ± 12.36
IgE/IgG4 ratio	0.28 ± 0.34	0.12 ± 0.19 ($p<0.025$)

Discussion

Our studies with ovalbumin as a model could not show a strong correlation between in vitro testing and oral provocation. Neither specific serum IgE, IgG1, IgG4 antibodies nor ovalbumin-induced histamine release from mixed leukocytes could predict a clinically relevant sensitization to ovalbumin. Only the IgE/IgG4 ratio different significantly between the two groups of symptomatically and asymptomatically sensitized children. The positive correlation between serum IgE antibodies to ovalbumin and the data on histamine release confirm that serum IgE antibodies correspond to the amount of IgE on basophils [18]. Our results are in accordance with the data of HILL [8] and SAMPSON [16], who also found that neither laboratory tests nor skin test could predict the clinical relevance of food allergy. Other authors, however, have reported a strong correlation between skin test results and positive oral challenge [3, 19, 20] and between histamine release, skin test and RAST results in egg-allergic patients [4]. The discrepancy between in vitro and in vivo data may be due to the fact that different effector cells are involved: basophil sensitivity and serum IgE do not necessarily correlate with mast cell sensitivity of skin, intestine or bronchus, we chose the model of immediate hypersensitivity to ovalbumin because it is easy to study in a rather standardized way.

Although the measurement of IgE and IgG subclass antibodies and the ovalbumin-induced histamine release may be of diagnostic value, only the oral provocation test can confirm the clinical relevance of hypersensitivity to food. However, symptoms to oral provocation are difficult to score since, for example, responses such as slight rashes, itching, nausea, headache and so-called tension fatigue still rely on patient's subjective assessment. It would be very useful to establish methods for quantification of allergic reactions after food challenge. Measuring gastrointestinal permeability with differently sized polyaethyleneglycoles [6] or with lactulose and mannitol [5] after oral provocation and the assessment of mediators or their metabolites (e.g. methyl-histamine) in plasma or urine may be good approaches to diagnose food allergy in a more rational way.

References

1. Anet J, Bach JF, Baker RS, Barnett D, Burley RW, Howden MEH (1985) Allergens in white and yolk of hen's egg. Int Arch Allergy Appl Immunol 77:364–371
2. Bock SA, May CD (1983) Adverse reactions to food caused by sensitivity. In: Middleton E, Reed CF, Ellis E (eds) Allergy - principles and practice, 2nd edn, vol 2. Mosby, St Louis, pp 1415ff chap 64
3. Bock SA, Lee W, Remigio LK, May CD (1978) Studies of hypersensitivity reaction to foods in infants and children. J Allergy Clin Immunol 62:327
4. Clinton PM, Kemeny DM, Amlot P, Urbanek R, Lessof MH (1986) Histamine release from peripheral blood leukocytes in egg allergic patients. Clin Allergy 16:345–354
5. Dupont C, Molkhou P, Dehennin L (1987) Diagnosis of food allergy by measurement of intestinal permeability in children with atopic dermatitis. Forty-third annual meeting of the American Academy of Allergy and Immunology, Washington D.C., 19–25 Februar
6. Fälth-Magnussen K, Kjellman NIM, Odelram H, Dundqvist T, Magnussen KE (1986) Gastrointestinal permeability in children with cow's milk allergy: effect of milk challenge and sodium cromoglycate as assessed with polyethylene-glycols (PEG 400, PEG 1000). Clin Allergy 16:543–551
7. Hattevig G, Kjellman B, Johannson SGO, Björksten B (1984) Clinical symptoms and IgE responses to common food proteins in atopic and healthy children. Clin Allergy 14:551–559
8. Hill DJ, Davidson GP, Cameron DJS, Barnes GC (1979) The spectrum of cow's milk allergy in childhood. Acta Paediatr Scan 68:847–852
9. Hoffman DR (1983) Immunochemical identification of allergens in egg white. J Allergy Clin Immunol 71:481
10. Kemeny DM, Urbanek R, Richards D, Greenall C (1987) Development of a semiquantitative enzyme-linked immunosorbent assay (ELISA) for detection of human IgG sublass antibodies. J Immunol Methods 96:47
11. Langeland T (1982) A clinical and immunological study of allergy to hen's egg white II. Antigen's in hen's egg white studied by immunoelectrophoresis (CIE). Allergy 37:323–333
12. Langeland T (1982) A clinical and immunological study of allergy to hen's egg white III. Allergens in hen's egg white studied by crossed radio-immunoelectrophoresis (CRIE). Allergy 37:521–530
13. Langeland T, Harbitz O (1983) A clinical and immunological study of allergy to hen's egg white IV. Purification and identification of a major allergen (antigen 22) in hen's egg white. Allergy 38:131–139
14. Maasch HJ, Fischer B, Wahl R, Wahn U (1984) Comparison of histamine release assay and RAST inhibition as tools for allergen extract standardization. Int Arch Allergy Appl Immunol 73:314–320
15. Metcalfe DD (1984) Food hypersensitivity. J Allergy Clin Immunol 73 (6):749–762
16. Sampson HA (1983) Role of immediate food hypersensitivity in the pathogenesis in atopic dermatitis. J Allergy Clin Immunol 71:473
17. Siraganian R (1974) An automated continuous flow system for the extraction and fluorometric analysis of histamine. Anal Biochem 57:393

18. Conroy MC, Adkinson NF, Lichtenstein LM (1977) Measurements of IgE- and anti-IgE-induced histamine release. J Immunol 118 (4):1317ff
19. Atikins AM, Steinberg SS, Metcalfe DD (1985) Evaluation of immediate adverse reaction to foods in adult patients, I Correlation of demographic laboratory and prick test data with response to controlled oral challenge. J Allergy Clin Immunol 348–355
20. May CD (1976) Objective clinical and laboratory studies of immediate hypersensitivity reactions to foods in asthmatic children. J Allergy Clin Immunol 58:500

Modifications of Intestinal Permeability to Large Molecules During Oral Provocation Tests in Children with Cow's Milk Sensitive Enteropathy and Atopic Dermatitis

C. Dupont, E. Barau and P. Molkhou

Introduction

The gut is characterized by a certain degree of leakiness, as a result of which molecules and macromolecules that are not actively absorbed may permeate passively through the intestinal wall. The degree of leakiness in, or rate of permeation across, the intestinal wall depends upon many factors, including the size of the molecule and the state of the mucosa [9, 15]. Practical methods to measure this permeability of the mucosa to molecules and macromolecules have been developed, based on measurement of the urinary excretion of orally absorbed non-metabolizable markers. The use of two probe molecules of different molecular sizes, such as mannitol and lactulose, exploits the principle of differential absorption, namely that the two markers behave similarly in all respects except in their rate of permeation across the mucosa. Expressing the relative rates of urinary excretion of the markers as a ratio thus allows the researcher to overcome the effects of the many non-relevant variables that may influence individual markers [10] and to compare results of repeat procedures performed under different clinical conditions. The aim of this study was to use a non-invasive technique to detect the food-induced alterations of mucosal integrity under conditions of cow's milk protein sensitive enteropathy (CMPSE) and atopic dermatitis (AD). The relationships of these conditions to food allergy, although still controversial, have been widely substantiated [2, 4, 13, 17, 20, 22].

We developed a protocol according to which intestinal permeability was evaluated in basal conditions (fasting test) and during concomitant ingestion of offending food (provocation test). This method allowed us to detect in hypersensitive patients the food-induced hyperpermeability of the large molecule lactulose as compared to that of mannitol and to ascertain a food-induced rise in the lactulose/mannitol urinary ratio [1].

Subjects and Methods

Twenty-five normal young children (aged from 6 months to 14 years) were used as controls. All were explored for poor growth and had a biopsy which revealed normal intestinal mucosa. None exhibited any gastro-intestinal or skin disease. In 7 infants (6 months to 2 years) CMPSE was clinically confirmed by the positivity of three milk challenge tests and in four of them by the presence of anti-cow's milk protein specific IgE (RAST, Pharmacia). All were studied after an exclusion diet lasting at least 3 months. Twenty-two children (6 months to 16 years) had AD. Of these, 13 had clinically confirmed (through improvement of skin lesions on excusion diet) and/or biologically confirmed (positive RAST and/or positive prick test in 9 out of 13) features of allergy to one or several foods: milk (6), egg (5), beef (1) or orange (1). These children were at the time of the test under exclusion diet for the related food antigen. For others, food allergy either was not clinically demonstrated or was being currently explored at the time of the study. Prick tests were performed with allergens purchased from Stallergens (France).

On the morning following an overnight fast of at least 6 h and after voiding and discarding overnight urine, the subjects were given a mixture of 10% mannitol aqueous solution (Pharmacie Centrale des Hôpitaux, Paris) and 65% lactulose aqueous solution (Duphalac, Duphar, France) at a dosage of 0.1 g/kg body weight for each sugar. During the following 5 h, all urine, including that passed at the end of the 5-h period, was collected, with merthiolate as a preservative.

For the fasting test, the solution of markers was given alone, subjects being allowed only glucose water during the 3rd, 4th and 5th hours of urine collection. For the provocation test, the solution of markers was given in mixture with food. Milk (50 ml) was given to children with CMPSE. Children with AD were given either 50 ml milk, half-egg, or 50 ml orange juice when these were clinically and/or biologically suggested to be responsible for the exacerbation of lesions. The same foods were given to controls. The volume of urine was measured, and aliquots were stored frozen. Samples were analysed later for mannitol and lactulose content by gas chromatography, as described previously [6].

Results were expressed as proportion of the oral lactulose to mannitol urinary excretion ratio (L/M ratio). For the provocation test, the L/M ratio was expressed by comparison to that of the fasting test – provocation L/M ratio to fasting L/M ratio (P/F). In children with CMPSE or AD, a provocation test with food was considered positive when P/F was more than 2 SD above the level in controls.

Results

In control children, the fasting L/M ratio (Fig. 1) was 2.73±0.70% (mean ±SD); this resulted from mean mannitol and lactulose urinary clearances of 16.30±5.77% and 0.33±0.10%, respectively (Table 1). Provocation tests (Fig. 2) performed in 11 cases (8 milk, 2 egg, 1 orange) resulted in a slight but non-significant decrease in the L/M ratio as compared to fasting test; P/F was 0.83±0.19.

In patients with CMPSE under exclusion diet, fasting L/M ratios were comparable to those of controls (Fig. 1; Table 1); only one value out of seven was 2 SD higher than the mean among controls. Milk ingestion (Fig. 2) induced a consistent rise in the L/M ratio; P/F was 3.57±3.47 ($p<0.02$, as compared with controls). This modification was due to a three-fold increase in lactulose urinary clearance ($p<0.05$, as compared to fasting value).

Table 1. Mannitol and lactulose urinary excretions after ingestion of 0.1 g/kg weight in control, CMPSE and AD patients in fasting conditions (fasting test) and with concomittant ingestion of offending food (provocation test)

	Mannitol urinary clearance (%)	Lactulose urinary clearance (%)	L/M (%)	P/F (%)
Controls ($n=25$)				
Fasting test	16.30± 5.77	0.33±0.10	2.73±0.70	
Provocation test ($n=11$)	12.60± 7.60	0.34±0.18	2.29±0.66	0.83±0.19
CMPSE ($n=7$)				
Fasting test	15.35± 6.03[a]	0.41±0.14[a]	2.63±1.28[a]	
Provocation test	14.71± 6.60[c]	1.02±0.69[d]	7.22±3.58[d]	3.57±3.48[b]
AD: normal fasting test ($n=13$)				
Fasting test	15.01± 7.70	0.31±0.15	2.37±0.79	
Provocation test	15.88±11.47[c]	0.50±0.31[d]	4.47±4.03[d]	1.76±1.23[b]
AD: abnormal fasting test ($n=9$)				
Fasting test	15.42± 8.04	0.97±0.51	6.91±3.30	
Provocation test	19.65± 7.97[c]	0.74±0.33[c]	5.27±3.32[c]	0.81±0.57[a]

L/M, ratio of lactulose to mannitol urinary clearance; P/F, ratio of provocation L/M ratio to fasting L/M ratio.
[a] Not significant, compared to controls.
[b] $p<0.05$, compared to controls.
[c] Not significant, compared to fasting value.
[d] $p<0.05$, compared to fasting value.

In children with AD, the fasting L/M ratio exhibited substantial variance, with a mean value significantly higher than that in controls: 4.23±3.12% ($p<0.02$). An L/M ratio 2 SD higher than the mean of controls was found in nine children (41%); this appeared to be due only to increased urinary clearance of lactulose: 0.97±0.51% versus 0.33±0.10% ($p<0.001$, as compared to controls). Provocation test results differed according to those of the fasting test. In 13 children with a normal fasting L/M ratio, provocation with milk (8), egg (4) or orange (1) induced a significant rise in the L/M ratio, with a P/F of 1.76±1.23 ($p<0.05$, as compared to controls). This, again, was related to an increased lactulose urinary clearance (Table 1). In nine children with an increased fasting L/M ratio, provocation with milk (6), egg (2) or beef (1) did not significantly alter the L/M ratio, with a P/F of 0.81±0.57. A positive provocation test (i.e. P/F>1.21) was found in 9/13 children with a normal fasting L/M ratio and 2/9 children with an increased fasting L/M ratio. In patients with AD related to a documented food allergy and who were tested with the offending food, the provocation

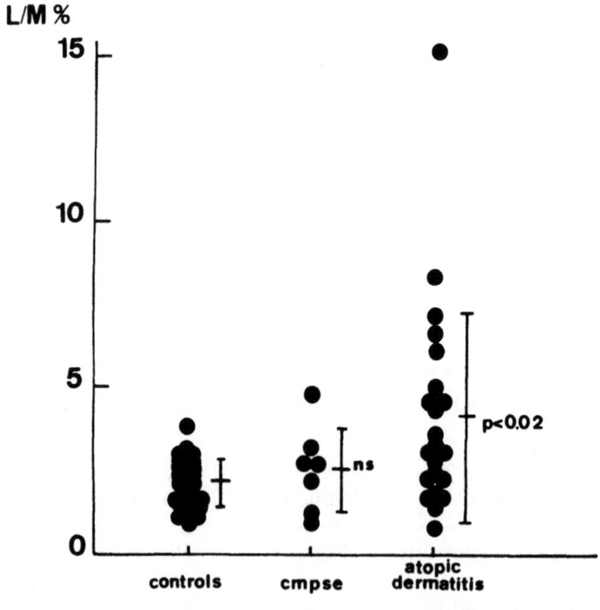

Fig. 1. Lactulose/mannitol urinary ratio (*L/M %*) after ingestion during fasting of 0.1 g/kg mannitol and lactulose in 25 control children, 7 children with CMPSE undergoing exclusion diet, and 22 children with AD (*p* refers to controls)

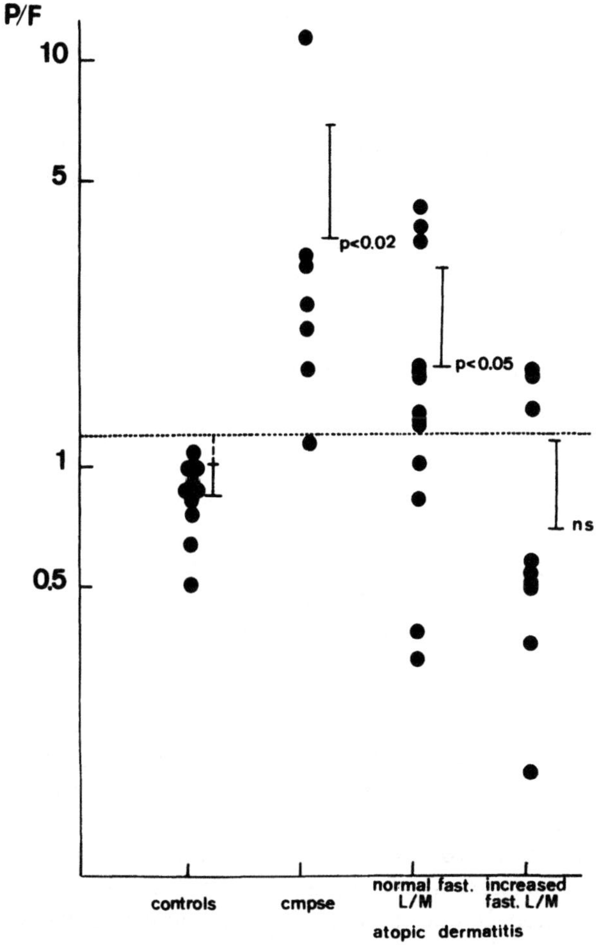

Fig. 2. Ratio of provocation L/M to fasting L/M ratio (*P/F*) after ingestion of 0.1 g/kg mannitol and lactulose together with milk in 7 patients with CMPSE and with milk, egg, orange or beef in 11 controls and 22 children with AD. *Dotted line* indicates mean + 2 SD of controls; above this value, provocation test is considered positive (*p* refers to controls)

test was positive in 6/7 cases with a normal fasting L/M ratio and in 1/6 with an increased fasting L/M ratio. An abnormal fasting L/M ratio and/or positive provocation test was found in 12/13.

Discussion

Comparative measurement of the urinary excretion of orally absorbed non-metabolizable sugars of different molecular sizes allows one to detect alterations in intestinal permeability under various pediatric intestinal conditions, such as coeliac disease and inflammatory bowel disease [5, 7, 16, 18]. Comparing urinary excretion of mannitol, a marker of small molecule absorption, and of lactulose, a marker of larger molecule absorption, was previously documented to be a good tool in the diagnosis of food allergy in adults [1]. This study is, to our knowledge, the first to make a systematic comparison of provocation test data to fasting test data in a pediatric population.

In controls, the L/M ratio during fasting appeared remarkably similar to that recorded in previous studies [18]. Concomitant ingestion of food induced a non-significant decrease in the L/M ratio, likely due to a decrease in the osmolarity of the mixture, leading to a decrease of the transmucosal passage of lactulose compared to mannitol [15].

In children with CMPSE, studied after a 3-month exclusion diet, the mean fasting L/M ratio was comparable to that in controls, probably reflecting mucosal integrity [21]. An L/M ratio 2 SD higher than the mean in controls was found in one child whose CMPSE had been diagnosed on failure to thrive, associated with partial villous atrophy. At the time of the study, clinical symptoms had resolved following exclusion diet, but intestinal biopsy revealed a persistent inflammatory process of the submucosa, together with a normal villous height.

In the provocation test with milk, the L/M ratio exhibited a three-fold increase, which appeared to be due mainly to a rise in lactulose excretion. In one child P/F remained under the value (1.21) which was considered, based on control data, as the criterion for positivity of the provocation test. This corroborates the findings in a previously published [10] series of three children with CMPSE; in two of these milk induced a two-fold rise in the lactulose/rhamnose ratio whereas in the other, who exhibited a mildly increased lactulose/rahmnose fasting ratio, milk induced no change.

In infants with CMPSE, the provocation test with milk was shown to induce a local reaginic reaction associated with villous height reduction and connective tissue oedema [21]. It is thus likely that these changes are responsible for the increased leakiness of intestinal mucosa to lactulose, which is thought to permeate across intestinal mucosa predominantly via the intercellular spaces and at extrusion zones at the villous tips [15]. In this process the role of the local release of allergy mediators remains speculative.

As regards AD, the results appeared less clear-cut. The fasting L/M ratio was either within the normal range or higher than 2 SD of the mean among controls, with a mean significantly higher than that of controls; this was related to an increased lactulose urinary clearance. This corroborates previous studies reporting an increased intestinal permeability in eczematous children as studied with polyethyleneglycol [12], lactulose and rhamnhose [8, 10, 19] or ^{51}Cr-labelled EDTA [11] and is likely to indicate, at least in some children, the presence of small-intestinal mucosal abnormalities. These are usually not gross histopathological alterations, as demonstrated in a previous morphological study of the jejunum in children with eczema due to food allergy [14] and in the five personal observations in which biopsies were performed. Indeed, minimal changes were seen in four of our cases with a mild, moderate lymphocytic infiltrate and sometimes with venous congestion. Focal villous atrophy was associated with inflammation in only one child with multiple food allergies, who also exhibited the highest L/M ratio of our series (15%), a value comparable to those observed in active coeliac disease [7].

In contrast to the case of children with CMPSE, those with AD did not exhibit a consistent increase in the L/M ratio in provocation tests. It is remarkable that a mean P/F significantly higher than that in controls was observed only in patients with a normal fasting L/M ratio. In these, 9 of 13 exhibited a positive food challenge in the intestinal permeability test, as opposed to 2 of 9 in the group of patients with an increased fasting L/M ratio. This difference raises a concern regarding the cause of the fasting hyperpermeability to lactulose. To some authors this seems to reflect a primary abnormality typically present at birth [23] and falling to "adult" values by the 9th day of life [3]. However, as Pike [19] has indicated, it is more likely that food allergy is the cause of this intestinal hyperpermeability. In this hypothesis, intestinal stimulation by allergens not withdrawn from the diet results in constant intestinal morphological or functional alterations. These food-induced alterations, with a resulting fasting hyperpermeability, may blunt the modifications induced by food allergens during provocations procedures.

In this respect, it is noteworthy that in children with AD and confirmed food allergy a positive provocation test with the recognized food antigen was found in 6 of 7 cases when the fasting L/M ratio was normal as compared to only 1 of 6 when the fasting L/M ratio was increased. It is our impression that the normal L/M ratio among the former reflects an appropriate withdrawal of the offending food, thus allowing a correct evaluation of food-induced hyperpermeability to lactulose in the challenge test. The latter group, on the other hand, was likely to be composed of children for whom food restriction was not appropriate. Further work is needed to clarify this crucial point.

In conclusion, our work demonstrates that comparing urinary excretion of mannitol and lactulose in basal conditions and after oral challenge with food is a useful tool in the diagnosis of a well-documented food allergy such as CMPSE. Our data also strongly support the involvement of food allergy in AD and indicate that studying intestinal permeability by means of provocation procedures may prove useful in the dietary management of this skin disease.

References

1. Andre C (1986) Allergie alimentaire. Diagnostic objectif et test de l'efficacité thérapeutique par mesure de la perméabilité intestinale. Presse Méd 15:105-108
2. Atherton DJ, Sewell M, Soothill JF, Wells RS, Chilvers CED (1978) A double-blind controlled crossover trial of an antigen avoidance diet in atopic eczema. Lancet 1:401-403
3. Beach RC (1984) Changes in gastro-intestinal permeability in the human neonate. MD Thesis, University of London, London, pp 145-158
4. Businco L, Businco E, Cantani A, Galli E, Infussi R, Benicori N (1982) Results of a milk and/or egg free diet in children with atopic dermatitis. Allergol Immunopathol 10:283-285
5. Cobden I, Dickinson RJ, Rothwell J, Axon ATR (1978) Intestinal permeability assessed by the excretion ratio of two molecules results in celiac disease. Br Med J ii:1060-1063
6. Dupont C, Barau E, Dehennin L, Molkhou P (1987) Mesure de la perméabilité intestinale aux sucres: application au diagnostic de la maladie coeliaque et de l'entéropathie aux protéines du lait de vache. Pathol Biol 35:1179-1182
7. Dupont C, Dehennin L, Navarro J, Canlorbe P (1987) Identification des syndromes de malabsorption par mesure de la perméabilité intestinale. Son application à la maladie coeliaque de l'enfant. Presse Méd 16:778
8. Du Mont GCL, Beach RC, Menzies IS (1984) Gastrointestinal permeability in food-allergic eczematous children. Clin Allergy 14:55-59
9. Ford RPK, Menzies IS, Phillips AD, Walker-Smith JA, Turner MW (1985) Intestinal sugar permeability: relationship to diarrhoeal disease and small bowel morphology. J Pediatr Gastroenterol Nutr 4:568-574
10. Ford RPK, Walker-Smith JA (1986) Food hypersensitivity and gut permeability. Frontiers of Gastrointestinal Research 13:69-81
11. Forget P, Sodoyez-Goffaux F, Zappitelli A (1985) Permeability of the small intestine to ^{51}Cr EDTA in children with acute gastroenteritis or eczema. J Pediatr Gastroenterol Nutr 4:393-396

12. Jackson PG, Lessof MH, Baker RWR, Ferrett J, McDonald DM (1981) Intestinal permeability in patients with eczema and food allergy. Lancet i:1285–1286
13. Juto P, Engberg S, Wimberg J (1978) Treatment of infantile atopic dermatitis with a strict elimination diet. Clin Allergy 8:493–500
14. McCalla F, Savilahti E, Perkkio M, Kuitunen P, Backman A (1980) Morphology of the jejunum in children with eczema due to food allergy. Allergy 35:563–571
15. Menzies IS (1983) Transmucosal passage of inert molecules in health and disease. In: Skadhauge E, Heintze K (eds) Intestinal absorption and secretion. MTP Press, London, pp 527–543
16. Menzies IS, Laker MF, Pounder R (1975) Abnormal permeability to sugars in villous atrophy. Lancet ii:1107–1109
17. Molkhou P, Waguet JC (1981) Food allergy and atopic dermatitis in children: treatment with oral sodium cromoglycate. Ann Allergy 47:173–175
18. Pearson ADJ, Eastham EJ, Laker MF, Craft AW, Nelson R (1982) Intestinal permeability in children with Crohn's disease and celiac disease. Br Med J 285:20–21
19. Pike MG, Heddle RJ, Boulton P, Turner MW, Atherton DJ (1986) Increased intestinal permeability in atopic eczema. J Invest Dermatol 86:101–104
20. Sampson HA (1983) Role of immediate food hypersensitivity in the pathogenis of atopic dermatitis. J Allerg Clin Immunol 71:473–480
21. Shiner M, Ballard J, Smith ME (1975) The small-intestinal mucosa in cow's milk allergy. Lancet i:136–140
22. Van Asperen PP, Lewis M, Rogers M, Kemp AS, Thompson S (1983) Experience with an elimination diet in children with atopic dermatitis. Clin. Allergy 13:479–485
23. Weaver LT, Laker MF, Nelson R, Lucas A (1987) Milk feeding and changes in intestinal permeability and morphology of the newborn. J Pediatr Gastroenterol Nutr 6:351–358

Whole Cow's Milk Versus Hydrolysed Infant Formulae: Analysis of Systemic Immune Responses and Antigenic Cross-Reactivities

S. Strobel and L. M. Fairclough

Introduction

There is no doubt that breast feeding is the most natural, hygienic, psychosocially important and least expensive way of feeding the young infant. Despite unequivocal advantages of breast feeding the young infant, cow's milk based formulae or other xenogeneic feeds (e.g. soya and pasteurised fortified goat's milk) are considered safe alternatives in the European setting and will certainly be used in future as they have been for over 80 years. The most commonly reported adverse clinical effects of cow's milk feeds are diarrhoea, vomiting and also failure to thrive, which is frequently due to an enteropathy. About 2% of infants suffer from more or less serious side effects of milk-containing feeds.

These side effects were reported as soon as cow's milk was introduced on a larger scale. Since then the available milk formulae have been adapted to meet the baby's nutritional requirements and have been "humanised", that is, adapted to levels of nutrients and vitamines found in breast milk. (Recommendations have been published by the Nutrition Committee of the European Society of Paediatric Gastroenterology and Nutrition [1, 2]). However, adaptation of these infant formulae to meet the baby's nutritional requirements has not overcome the major immunological disadvantage of such practice: the administration of *foreign* macromolecular antigens at a time when physiological parameters of the neonatal gut and gut-associated lymphoid tissues are inexperienced or immature.

Reduction of the Antigenicity of Cow's Milk

Since cow's milk allergy or food-allergic diseases, generally, are a feature of infancy, it seemed logical to reduce the allergenicity of cow's milk proteins by a variety of different technical procedures. Hydrolysates have been manufactured for over 40 years using two main technologies: heat denaturation and/or enzymatic (tryptic) hydrolysis [3]. Both procedures are generally used to yield an optimal balance between palatibility and residual antigenicity. Simplifying, it can be said that a decrease in molecular weight of the remaining peptides – and most likely also a decrease in their inherent immunogenicity – is accompanied by a decrease in palatibility. Pure amino acid mixtures are not only of poor sensory quality but may also be of inferior nutritional quality [4].

Reducing the sensitising (immunising) capacity of a protein by digestion, and thus reducing the size of the residual peptide, forms the basis for manufacturing protein hydrolysates. The immunochemical characteristics of these formulae, and with them their sensitising capacity, varies considerably and are dependent on the protein source, extent of hydrolysis, post-hydrolysis processing and removal of the peptidases used during the manufacturing process. Physical properties and antigenic potential of milk proteins, clinical experience in treating (and challenging) milk-sensitive patients and the results of skin tests with some cow's milk proteins have led to the assumption that the allergenic potential is different for various cow's milk proteins. Results of two studies are summarised in Table 1, with β-lactoglobulin (BLG) leading (82%), followed by the caseins and α-lactalbumin (43%, 41%, respectively) [5, 6].

It is almost impossible to yield uncontaminated BLG or α-casein preparations, and some of the discrepant results may be explained by this fact. If, for example, BLG, the most stable whey protein, is heated in the presence of caseins, it is coprecipitated with the caseins [7]. Caseins are of low ordered structure and resist heat treatment for prolonged

Table 1. Skin test results of cow's milk allergic individuals to isolated cow's milk proteins

Protein	Responses [5]	Protein	Responses [6]
Casein	34 (57) %	β-Lactoglobulin	82%
α-Lactalbumin	22 (54) %	α-Lactalbumin	43%
β-Lactoglobulin	20 (66) %	Casein	41%
Bovine serum albumin	21 (54) %	Bovine γ-globulin	27%
		Bovine serum albumin	18%

Figures in parentheses indicate the percentage of skin test positive children to one or more cow's milk proteins who developed clinical symptoms when challenged with the isolated proteins ($n = 45$).

times. The highly structured globular whey proteins such as BLG, bovine serum albumin (BSA) and bovine IgG are easily heat coagulated and irreversibly denatured [8]. All cow's milk proteins are potential immunogens due to a great extent of sequence *non*-homology between human and bovine proteins.

As pointed out above, heat treatment does mainly affect whey proteins but not caseins. These must be degraded by proteolytic cleavage with endopeptidases (trypsin, chymotrypsin, papain and others). Progressive hydrolysis eliminates sequential (non-conformational) determinants. The residual antigenicity and thus potential allergenicity (triggering of an allergic hypersensitivity reaction) is dependent on the food-processing technologies applied, and these are often a well-kept secret of the manufacturer.

Analysis of Immunogenicity and Cross-Reactivities of Hydrolysed Formulae

There are no clear instructions for the analysis or comparison of hydrolysed infant feeds since most of these are not considered as *prescribable drugs* in the original sense. Animal models such as the guinea-pig anaphylaxis test [9] or the anaphylaxis test described in the United States Pharmacopia for "hydrolysates to be used for injection" [10] have been applied, as well as competitive radioimmunoassays. These assay systems vary considerably in their sensitivity, with ranges from milligram to microgram equivalents of starting cow's milk proteins.

Most test systems have the following disadvantages in common: (a) focus on anaphylactic responses (IgE) only; (b) restriction to only three (BLG, casein, BSA) of more than 40 cow's milk proteins; (c) no investigation of antigenicity and cross-reactivity of cow's milk and its breakdown products (peptides) in a complete cross-over design (see Fig. 2); and (d) failure to asses cell-mediated immune responses which seem to be under different immunological control (see below) [11].

Investigations of cross-reactivities between antibody responses and cell-mediated immunity induced by the *whole molecule* as compared to the *hydrolysate* are of particular importance. Such focus is even more important if the hydrolysate formula is to be used not only prophylactically but for the *treatment* of children with cow's milk protein-sensitive diseases such as enteropathy, anaphylaxis, eczema or migraine (Fig. 1).

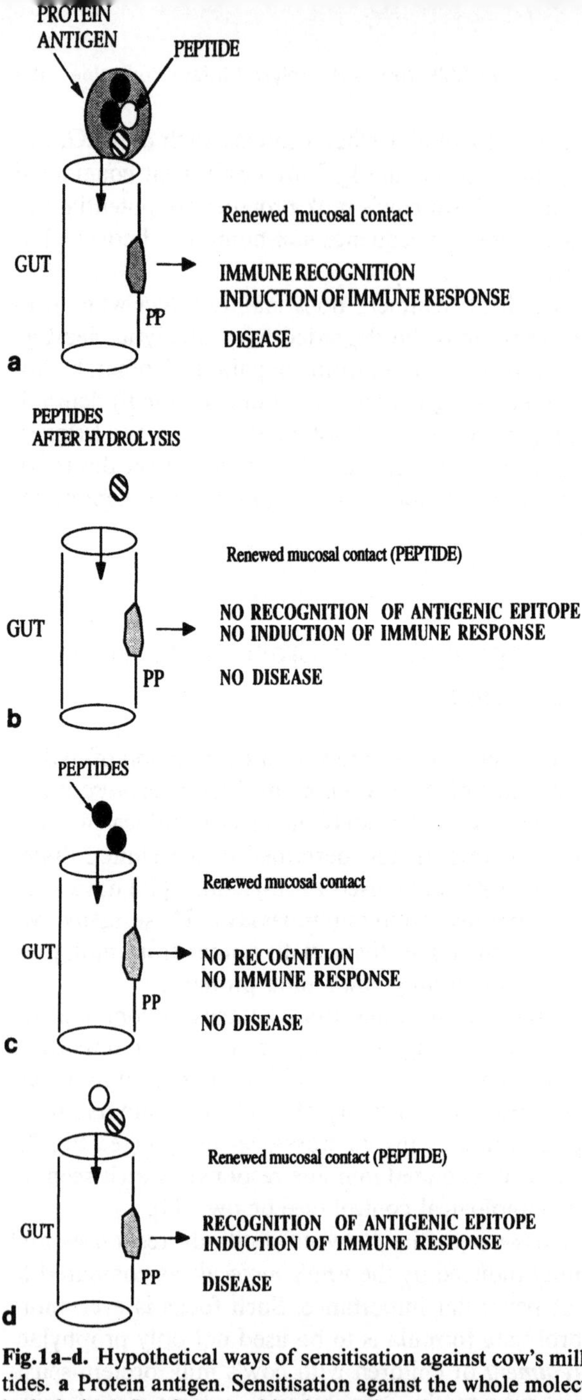

Fig. 1 a–d. Hypothetical ways of sensitisation against cow's milk proteins and/or peptides. **a** Protein antigen. Sensitisation against the whole molecule. **b–d** Peptides after hydrolysis. **b** Previous sensitisation against the whole molecule peptides are not recognised; no disease. **c** Enteral exposure to a small peptide may not sensitise against itself or the intact protein molecule. **d** Previous sensitisation against the whole molecule including sensitisation against epitopes displayed by a peptide

Experimental Design, Materials and Methods

We will briefly describe an experimental model [12] which was used to investigate the immunogenicity and cross-reactivity of a newly developed hydrolysed infant formula compared with a standard cow's milk formula and already available "low-allergenic" (hydrolysed) infant feeds.

The general study design is outlined in Fig. 2. Animals (mice) were immunised with complete Freund's adjuvant (CFA) mixed in equal volumes with the whole protein formula, constitutents of the hydrolysed formulae and with the final hydrolysed infant formula as given to the infant. Substances used in this study were (the letter in parentheses representing the short-hand notation):

Aptamil (Milupa), cow's milk formula (A)
Hyprol 8009, pure soy/beef hydrolysate, used in W 237 and Pregomin (B)
W 237, a developmental batch of Pregomin (C)
Pregomin (Milupa), soy/beef hydrolysate (D)
Pregestimil (Mead Johnson), casein hydrolysate (E)
Corn and potato starch, constituent of W 237 (C) and Pregomin (F)
Alfaré (DS 24, Nestlé), whey protein hydrolysate (G)
Nutramigen (Bristol Myers), casein hydrolysate (H)

Antibody responses and delayed hypersensitivity reaction against the immunising antigen and the different recall antigens were measured by a sensitive enzyme-linked immunosorbent assay (ELISA) technique and by assessing cell mediated immune responses by measuring the specific skin footpad increments 24 h after antigen injection in previously immunised animals. Groups of control animals were immunised either with CFA and saline or with CFA and the test antigens; they were injected with saline to detect non-specific responses. Statistical compari-

The immune responses of each experimental group immunised with *one* antigen are tested against *all* antigens.

IMMUNISE with antigen A in CFA

RECALL with A for immunogenicity
B
C
D etc. for

assessment of immunogenicity *and* cross reactivity

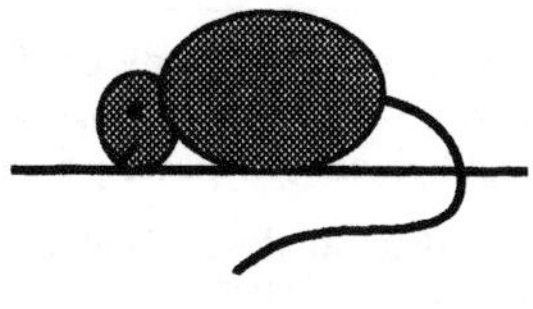

Fig. 2. General study design

son between groups (from six to eight animals per group) was performed with Student's *t* test using the Abstat computer program.

Results

Antibody Binding Assays (ELISA). The results demonstrate an unexpected finding. Antibodies raised against a cow's milk formula (A) bound (recognised) to epitopes displayed by peptides of hydrolysed formulae or to other constitutents of these hydrolysates (B-G) and to H (not used for immunisation) (Table 2). Antisera raised against B and G bound to wells coated with whole cow's milk proteins (A). Antisera raised against B-G did not bind to wells coated with antigens B-G. This was not due to the failure of these peptides to bind to the plastic wells since control experiments using radioactively labelled peptides confirmed their binding to the plastic surface.

One possible explanation for the inability to measure antibody responses against most of the hydrolysates could be the fact that these peptides act as *haptens* and are not large enough to elucidate an immune response without being coupled to a carrier protein. If cow's milk

Table 2. Immunogenicity and cross-reactivity: antibody responses

Coating antigens	Immunising antigens A	B	C	D	E	F	G
A	**+++**	**+**	0	0	0	0	**++**
B	**+**	**0**	0	0	0	0	0
C	**++**	0	**0**	0	0	0	0
D	**++**	0	0	**0**	0	0	0
E	**++**	0	0	0	**0**	0	0
F	**++**	0	0	0	0	**0**	0
G	**+**	0	0	0	0	0	**0**
H	**++**	0	0	0	0	0	0

Summary of antibody binding analysis (ELISA). Positive responses and results obtained with identical coating and immunising antigens (1^0 and 2^0 immunisation) are highlighted. For description of substances tested, see text.

Statistical analysis (2-tailed Student's *t* test):

+++ $p<0.001$
++ $p<0.01$
+ $p<0.05$
0 $p>0.05$

is used as an immunising agent, the specific antibodies produced may well have recognition sites for the epitopes displayed by the hydrolysed peptides. The observed cross-reactivity of antibodies raised against a cow's milk formula – which could be interpreted as a hapten-carrier model – to hydrolysed peptides would favour the latter explanation.

Cell-Mediated Immunity. A different pattern of responsiveness was seen when antigenicity and cross-reactivity of delayed hypersensitivity responses were assessed (Table 3). The results confirm the immunogenic nature of the non-hydrolysed formula (cow's milk) and the reduced immunogenicity of the hydrolysed formulae, however to a lesser extent than that seen for antibody responses. Animals immunised with antigens B and D, and more pronouncedly so when immunised with F and G, showed a positive skin test result ($p<0.05$ or <0.01). Other cross-reactivities are detailed in Table 3. The pattern of epitope recognition, which differs for the two limbs of immune response, stresses the necessity to investigate both humoral *and* cell-mediated immunity, both of which have been shown to be under different, as yet ill-defined, control mechanisms [12].

Table 3. Immunogenicity and cross-reactivity: cell-mediated immunity

Recall antigens	Immunising antigens A	B	C	D	E	F	G
A	+++	+	0	0	0	+	0
B	+	+	0	0	0	0	0
C	0	0	**0**	0	+	0	0
D	0	0	0	+	0	++	0
E	0	nd	0	0	**0**	nd	nd
F	+	nd	0	nd	0	+++	0
G	0	0	0	nd	++	0	++

Specific footpad increments 24 h after injection; primary immunisation and recall antigens as indicated. For description of substances tested, see text. Positive specific skin test responses and crossreactivities are highlighted. (Antigen H not tested).

Statistical analysis (2-tailed Student's *t* test):
+++ $p<0.001$
++ $p<0.01$
+ $p<0.05$
0 $p>0.05$
nd not investigated

Obvious ethical contraints prevent tests of the residual immunogenicity of an infant formula in children. Our experimental model has been successfully used to investigate immunogenicity and cross-reactivity of a hydrolysed formula for both limbs of the immune response and obviates potentially hazardous test procedures in children.

Conclusions

The results of this study may be summarised as follows:

1. Hydrolysed infant formulae are less immunogenic than currently available cow's milk formulae when introduced into the tissue of an experimental animal.
2. Immune responses to hydrolysates, however, can be elicited by hyperimmunisation techniques and differ for antibody and cell-mediated immune responses. These finding suggest that the immunological analyses of a hydrolysed infant formula must incorporate the assessment of antibody responses (e.g. IgG and IgE) and also of cell-mediated immune responses.
3. Antibodies raised against a cow's milk based formula recognise epitopes on hydrolysed peptides at various levels, dependent on the extent of hydrolysis.

On the basis of our observations obtained with the experimental model decribed here, it would seem possible that children who are highly allergic to cow's milk could still react to currently available hydrolysed infant formulae. It would seem much less likely that infants could be sensitised to cow's milk proteins after having received a hydrolysed formula. It is premature, however, to advocate the blanket use of hydrolysed formulae to prevent or reduce the incidence of cow's milk related diseases at this time. Clinical studies which address these important issues are currently under way.

Acknowledgement. L.F. gratefully acknowledges the support of Milupa AG, Friedrichsdorf/Ts, Federal Republic of Germany.

References

1. Nutrition Committee of the European Society of Paediatric Gastroenterology and Nutrition (1982) Guidelines on infant nutrition II. Recommendation for infant feeding. ESPGAN Committee on Nutrition. Acta Paedriatr Scand [Suppl] 302:1-27
2. Nutrition Committee of the European Society of Paediatric Gastroenterology and Nutrition (1987) Nutrition and feeding of preterm infants. ESPGAN Committe on Nutrition, B Wharton (ed). Acta Paedriatr Scand [Suppl] 336:1-14
3. Knights RJ (1985) Processing and evaluation of the antigenicity of protein hydrolysates. In: Lifshitz F, ed. Nutrition for special needs in infancy. Dekker, New York
4. Albinia JE, Jacobs DO, Melnik G, et al. (1985) Nitrogen utilisation from elemental diets. J Parent Enteral Nutr 9:189-195
5. Goldman AS, Anderson DW, Sellars WA, et al. (1963) Milk allergy. I. Oral challenge with milk and isolated milk proteins in allergic children. Pediatrics 32:425-443
6. Freier S, Kletter B, Lebenthal E, Griefman M (1969) Intolerance to milk protein. J Pediatr 75:623-631
7. Sawyer WH (1969) Complex between β-lactoglobulin and κ-casein. A review. J Dairy Sci 52:1347-1355
8. Jost R, Monti JC, Pahud JJ (1987) Whey protein allergenicity and its reduction by technological means. Food Technology 41:118-121
9. Anderson KJ, McLaughlan P, Devey ME, Coombs RRA (1979) Anaphylactic sensitivity of guinea pigs drinking different preparations of cow's milk and infant formulae. Clin Exp Immunol 35:454-461
10. Protein hydrolysate injection. In: The United States Pharmacopia XX, 1980, pp 687-688
11. Strobel S, Ferguson A (1987) Persistence of oral tolerance in mice is different for humoral and cellular immune responses. Immunology 60:317-318
12. Strobel S, Anderson DM, Ferguson A (1986) Immunogenicity and crossreactivity and nonspecific irritant properties of the exudate gums acacia, karaya, and tragacanth. Food Addit Contam 3:47-56

The Binding Capacity of IgE to Hypoallergenic Nutrients

C. P. Bauer

Introduction

Since publication of the research by CRONER [4], KJELLMAN [5], and DUCHATEAU et al. [6], one method of atopy prevention in infants is provided through an exclusive diet of breast-fed milk during the first 6 months of life. Medical observations suggest that early dietary contact with animal and plant protein may be responsible for the early development of atopic diseases in children of high-risk groups.

Especially for this reason, one currently tries to prohibit the intake of animal and plant proteins by newborn infants; experimentally, as an alternative to breast feeding, so-called hypoallergenic nutrients (hydrolysates) are being used. The raw material in the majority of these hypoallergenic diets is cow's milk or soya protein. A reduction of the allergen content of these raw materials is obtained by enzymically dividing the proteins. Nonallergens, however, can not be produced through hydrolysis; only hypoallergen nutrients can be produced in this way.

In our research we have attempted to examine the degree to which protein fractions are present as a nutritional component causing a specific IgE binding upon encountering the appropriate IgE antibody and are in this way identified as allergens by allergy sufferers; in addition, we have compared the probable IgE-binding capacity of this nutrient to that of mother's milk.

Methods

The research methods employed were the radioimmunosorbent test (RAST), gel electrophoresis, immune blotting, and the prick test. To identify specific IgE antibodies, we used RAST plates produced by Pharmacia. During the production of the plates, laboratory nutrition and mother's milk were consecutively put on paper plates. The mother's milk samples were taken from one mother who drank less than 0.25 l milk per day (M 20) and from a mother who drank at least 1.5 l milk per day (M 21). RAST plates with serum samples from children known to have cow's milk allergies were examined. The analysis was done in Phadebas RAST units (PRU; Table 1). The gel electrophoresis was conducted horizontally, and the BENGTSSON and EINARSSON [7, 8, 9] immune blotting modification was used.

The same serum samples (A and F) were used for both immune blotting and RAST examination as well as the patient serum sample (G). The prick test was conducted with each nutrient in the following fluid concentration: Beba-HA 13.2 %, dissolvable Humana HP 15.5%. We used a 0.9% NaCl solution as negative control and a histamine solution as positive control [1].

Table 1. IgE binding of five milk preparations in Phadebas RAST on incubation with sera from 12 patients with known specific IgE concentration against cow's milk (and three negative controls)

Serum	Cow's milk (PRU/ml)	Humana HP (PRU/ml)	Beba HA (PRU/ml)	Breast milk 20 (PRU/ml)	Breast milk 21 (PRU/ml)
1	>17.9	1.6	8.0	0.99	0.86
7	11.6	1.3	1.5	<0.35	<0.35
12	2.0	<0.35	0.36	<0.35	<0.35
13	4.5	<0.35	0.56	<0.35	<0.35
14	7.8	<0.35	0.35	<0.35	<0.35
15	5.8	<0.35	0.35	<0.35	<0.35
16	5.4	<0.35	1.1	0.77	0.83
A	2.1	0.82	0.65	0.56	0.62
F	5.6	0.88	1.7	0.56	0.76
B	15.2	1.2	1.7	0.49	0.56
C	3.0	<0.35	<0.35	1.2	0.87
D	4.8	1.6	1.2	0.78	0.75
Negative	<0.35	<0.35	<0.35	<0.35	<0.35
Negative	<0.35	<0.35	<0.35	<0.35	<0.35
Negative	<0.35	<0.35	<0.35	<0.35	<0.35

RAST classes
- 0: <0.35 PRU/ml
- 1: 0.35–0.7 PRU/ml
- 2: 0.7–3.5 PRU/ml
- 3: 3.5–17.5 PRU/ml
- 4: >17.5 PRU/ml

Results

The specific IgE antibodies were identified as positive in all the patients' serum samples examined, from patients known to have IgE antibodies to cow's milk (minimum RAST, 2) as well as in Beba-HA (RAST, 0.35 PRU/ml), with the exception of patient serum sample C. Six out of 12 serum samples in Humana HP were positive (RAST, 0.35 PRU), and the corresponding negative controls were all negative (0.35 PRU; Table 1).

Using gel elctrophoresis and Humana HP, shadows at less than 66000 daltons and protein band impressions were identified. Therefore, it is assumed that neither nutrient is completely hydrolysed, and that both contain IgE-bindable proteins. Both mother's milk and cow's milk showed a similar distribution of protein bands.

During the immune blotting (Fig. 1) molecule-sized IgE binding between 14000 and 40000 daltons were unquestionably identified, although the IgE bands varied from one patient serum to the other; IgE bindings above 60000 daltons were questionable. The hydrolysat nutrient did not cause nonspecific binding among the negative controls. Different IgE bindings resulted, both with mother's milk and in the negative controls, so that one might assume that nonspecific bindings are present as well. The results from immune blotting must be taken into consideration when interpreting the positive RAST results of mother's milk.

Patient numbers 11, 7, 12, 13, 14, 15, and 16 were given the skin test; their serum samples were also used during the RAST examination. Patients 17 and 18 were included in this stage of the examination, and number 19 was included as a negative control.

Four of the ten examined children (with known cow's milk allergies, RAST ≥ 2) showed positive reactions to the prick test with Beba HA, and four patients showed positive or slightly positive reactions to Humana HP (Fig. 1; Table 2).

Summary

Both of the new hypoallergic infant diets, Beba HA and Humana HP, contain protein fractions which, when correctly incubated with serum samples from patients allergic to cow's milk, resulted in a specific IgE binding. Accordingly, an allergic reaction could occur when patients who are allergic to cow's milk are given this diet. It has not yet been

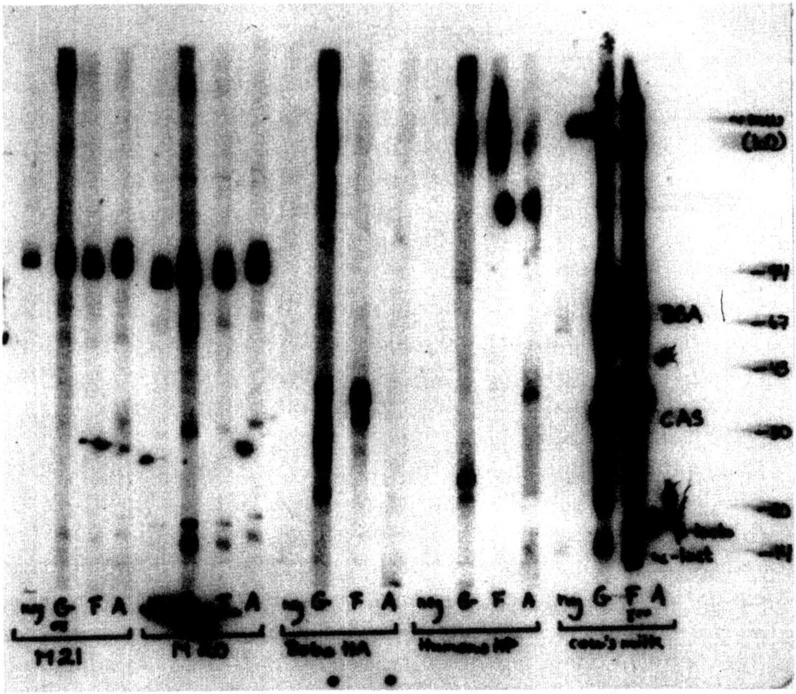

Fig. 1. Immunoblotting with five milk preparations with sera of three patients with cow's milk allergy G, F, A and one negative control. *M 21*, breast milk from a woman drinking at least 1.5 l milk per day; *M 20*, breast milk from a woman drinking less than 0.25 l milk per day

Table 2. Skin prick test with Humana HP (15.5%), Beba HA (13.2%) and cow's milk in nine patients with known cow's milk allergy (and one negative control)

Patient number	PRU/ml	Cow's milk	Humana HP	Beba HA	0.9% NaCl	Histamine
1	>17.9	++++	+++	+++	∅	+++
7	11.6	++++	++	+++	∅	+++
12	2.0	+++	∅	∅	∅	+++
13	4.5	+++	+	++	+	+++
14	7.8	+++	++	++	∅	+++
15	5.8	++++	++	+	∅	+++
16	5.4	+++	∅	+	+	+++
17	3.0	+++	∅	∅	∅	+++
18	2.8	+++	+	+	+	+++
19	<0.35	∅	∅	∅	∅	+++

established whether this diet could play a role in the prevention of atopy among neonates. It cannot be assumed that the protein fractions found in the hypoallergenic diets examined, which resulted in a specific IgE binding in already sensitized patients, would also lead to sensitization in high atopy risk-group neonates.

Acknowledgement. I would like to thank Mrs. A. BORGA, (Pharmacia, Sweden) for her support during the laboratory research.

References

1. Bauer CP, Krebs S, Loos, W (1985) Evaluation of cord-blood-IgE by an EIA. Ann Allergy 55:551
2. Bauer CP, Franz R, Belohradsky BH (1985) Cord-blood-IgE determination by enzyme-immuno-assay. Correlation between above normal IgE-values and lymphocyte populations. Pediatr Res 19:1119
3. Bauer CP, Schlemmer P, Franz R, Grübl H, Belohradsky BH, Emmrich P (1986) T-cell ratio in newborns and one year old children at risk of developing atopy. Pediatr Res 20:1039
4. Croner S, Kjellman M (1982) IgE-screening in 1701 newborn infants and the development of atopic disease during infancy. Arch Dis Child 57:364–368
5. Duchateau J, Casimir G (1983) Neonatal serum IgE concentrations as prediction of allergy. Lancet II:413
6. Saarinen UMA, et al. (1979) Prolonged breast-feeding as propohylaxis for atopic disease. Lancet II:163–166
7. Bengtsson A, Karlsson A, Rolfsen W, Einarsson R (1986) Detection of allergens mould and mite preparations by a nitrocellulose electroblotting technique. Int Arch Allergy Appl Immunol 90:383–390
8. Tovey ER, Baldo BA (1987) Characterisation of allergens by protein blotting. Electropohoresis 8:452–463

How Allergenic are "Hypoallergenic" Formulas?

S. Lau and U. Wahn

Immediate hypersensitivity reactions to cow's milk proteins can often be found in early childhood [3–5, 7, 11]. Cow's milk is the first protein-rich food that most infants receive after weaning. All the known antigens of cow's milk are proteins (Table 1). Cow's milk contains more than 25 distinct proteins that may act as antigens in man [1, 2, 6]. The most important allergens are casein and the whey proteins β-lactoglobulin, α-lactalbumin, bovine serum albumin (BSA) and immunoglobulin. Some 60%–80% of milk-allergic patients have serum IgE to β-lactoglobulin, 60% to casein, 50% to α-lactalbumin and BSA, and up to 40% to immunoglobulin [1, 2].

Table 1. Cow's milk proteins

Protein	MW	pI	% of total protein
Casein	20000–30000	3.7–6.0	82
β-Lactoglobulin	18000	5.3	9
α-Lactalbumin	14000	5.1	3
Serum albumin	67000	4.7	1
Immunoglobulin	160000	5.6–6.0	2

(From [6])

Table 2. Hydrolysed cow's milk formulas

Formula	Source	Processing
Formula A	Whey protein	Hydrolysis, heating
Formula B	Soy, bovine collagen	Hydrolysis, heating
Formula C	Casein	Hydrolysis, heating
Formula D	Soy, whey protein, bovine collagen	Hydrolysis, heating
Formula E	Whey protein	Hydrolysis, heating

Whey proteins are more heat labile than casein [1, 2, 6, 9]. In recent years so-called "hypoallergenic" formulas have been developed. These formulas are processed by heat and enzymatic hydrolysis, and the conformational and sequential structures are changed. The formulas contain peptides of lower molecular weight than the native protein source, which some authors think to be less immunogenic [6]. In Table 2 the protein sources and the processing of five formulas are shown.

Material and Methods

In our study we investigated 15 children with cow's milk allergy. Histamine release from washed leukocytes was performed, comparing the histamine release induced by cow's milk proteins with the release induced by the five formulas. The children were aged from 3 months to 5 years (mean, 18 months). They had serum IgE levels to cow's milk (radioallergosorbent test, RAST, $\geqslant 2$), positive history (type I reaction) and a significant ($>20\%$) histamine release to at least one of the proteins casein, β-lactoglobulin and α-lactalbumin. Ten children had atopic eczema, two had bronchial asthma, one had atopic eczema and bronchial asthma and two had gastrointestinal symtoms after milk ingestion. The histamine release assay was performed according to SIRAGANIAN [12]. After 90 min sedimentation in dextran the mixed leukocytes were incubated for 40 min (37 °C) with serial dilutions of casein, β-lactoglobulin, α-lactalbumin and five formulas: formulas A to E (0.0001–10 µg/ml). The histamine contents of the supernatants were measured fluorometrically [12]. The basophil sensitivity – Ag_{20}, i.e. the antigen concentration in micrograms required to release 20% of cellular histamine – was determined.

Negative controls were 28 atopic children without IgE to cow's milk protein who were investigated for histamine release to cow's milk proteins and the five formulas.

Results

Of the 15 children, 12 released histamine from washed leukocytes on incubation with casein, 6 with α-lactalbumin and 12 with β-lactoglobulin. Six were positive to all milk proteins and five released histamine to only one protein. The median threshold concentration for Ag_{20} was 1.55 µg/ml for casein, 0.34 µg/ml for α-lactalbumin and 0.6 µg/ml for β-lactoglobulin.

Nine of fifteen patients released histamine to at least one of the five formulas (formula A, 4/15; formula B, 4/15; C, 4/15; D, 4/4; E, 0/2). (Only four patients were tested for formula D, and only two were tested for formula E). None of the patients reacted to all the formulas. Onc patient reacted to four formulas, one to three formulas (A, B, D), two patients to two formulas (A+C, A+B) and five patients only to one formulas (two patients to formula C, two to formula D and one to B).

The median values (Ag_{20}) were 4.0 µg/ml for formula A, 3.3 µg/ml for B, 2.0 µg/ml for C and 1.25 µg/ml for D. The median values for AG_{20} were lower for cow's milk proteins than for formulas. These values, however, cannot actually by compared because, on one hand, the cow's milk proteins were used as a rather pure fraction, and, on the other, the formulas were used as a mixture of proteins, sugars and fat. One cannot, thus, compare molar concentrations of proteins (formula B cannot be compared, in any case, because its protein source is bovine collagen and soy).

Twenty-eight children without serum IgE to cow's milk were investigated for histamine release as a specificity control, and all reacted negatively to cow's milk and formula.

Discussion

Investigating 15 children sensitive to cow's milk with a positive histamine release from mixed leukocytes, we found in nine children also a positive histamine release to at least one of five tested formulas. Although the proteins of these formulas have been hydrolized and therefore contain peptides of lower molecular weight than the native protein source, the peptides still have allergenic potency and can be recognized by cell-bound IgE of an individual allergic to cow's milk. An exact comparison between threshold concentrations for milk proteins and formulas was not possible in this study. One can conclude that the formulas still contain epitopes of the native protein. Products with more than one protein source, such as formula D, seem to be more likely to induce histamine release than products derived from only one protein source. Although the 28 children not allergic to cow's milk did not react in the histamine release assay either to cow's milk or to formula (so that the assay procedure seems to be specific), it has not yet been proven whether the formulas may have osmotic [10] activity, which would be a nonspecific effect. Histamine release experiments in the absence of calcium must be performed to exclude this.

References

1. Aas K (1976) Common characteristics of major allergens. In: Johannsson SGO, Strandberg K (eds) Molecular and biological aspects of the acute allergic reaction. Plenum, New York, pp 3–19
2. Aas K (1978) What makes an allergen an allergen? Allergy 33:3–14
3. Anderson JA, Sogn DD (eds) (1984) Adverse reactions to foods. AAAI and NIAID Report, NIH Publication no 84-2442
4. Bock SA (1982) The natural history of food sensitivity. J Allergy Clin Immunol 69:173–177
5. Businco L, Benincori N, Cantani A (1984) Epidemiology, incidence and clinical aspects of food allergy. Ann Allergy 53:615–622
6. Gjesing B, Lowenstein H (1984) Immunochemistry of food antigens. Ann Allergy 53:602
7. Hattevig G, Kjellman B, Johannsson SGO, Björksten B (1984) Clinical symptoms and IgE responses to common food proteins in atopic and healthy children. Clin Allergy 14:559
8. Hill DJ, Davidson GP, Cameron DJS, Barnes GL (1979) The spectrum of cow's milk allergy in childhood. Acta Paediatr Scand 68:847–852
9. King TP (1976) Chemical and biological properties of some atopic allergens. Adv Immunol 23:77–105
10. Rimmer J, Bryant DH (1986) Effect of hypo- and hyper-osmolarity on basophil histamine release. Clin Allergy 16:221–230
11. Sampson HA (1983) Role of immediate hypersensitivity in the pathogenesis of atopic dermatitis. J Allergy Clin Immunol 71 (5):473–480
12. Siraganian R (1974) An automated continuous flow system for the extraction and fluorometric analysis of histamine. Anal Biochem 57:383

Experience with Hypoallergenic Formulas in the Treatment of Food Allergy in Infancy

R. M. Bertele-Harms and H. K. Harms

Food allergy manifests itself in infancy as a malabsorption syndrome following small-intestinal mucosal injury, caused by a complex immunological process, or it is an exclusively IgE-mediated allergy in which the morphology and function of the small intestinal mucosa is hardly affected, and malabsorption is not of primary significance. Consequently, the various treatment requirements of the dystrophic infant a few weeks old, who has not been breast fed and presents with malabsorption and damage to the mucosa, are higher and more complex than for the purely IgE-mediated form, for which a selective diet is normally sufficient.

The primary objective in dystrophic infants is to reestablish an anabolic situation through which the damaged mucosa has a real chance of repair. Since mucosa injury and malabsorption interfere with sufficient oral intake of calories at the beginning of treatment, a predominant parenteral nutrition, using a central venous catheter, is usually necessary. Nonetheless, a small amount of a suitable and easily absorbed food should always be applied orally from the beginning in order to make use of its local healing properties.

What is a suitable and easily absorbed food? The answer to this question can be derived from historical examples in the 1970s, from which we have learnt a great deal.

One of the earliest mistakes was to pay too little attention to the osmolarity of formulas. Figure 1 shows this in the example of an infant who was given an amino acid mixture together with carbohydrates and oil via a feeding tube. Following application of a 10% glucose solution, with an osmolarity of 555 mosmol/l, a strongly hyperosmotic solution was used, which osmotically exacerbated the diarrhoea. If a polysaccharide, e.g. maltodextrin or starch, had been applied instead, the osmolarity would have been markedly reduced. Nonetheless, the application of polysaccharides is not without problems, as shown in the treatment of acute enteritis by Sandhu et al. [2] and Meeuwisse [1]. The

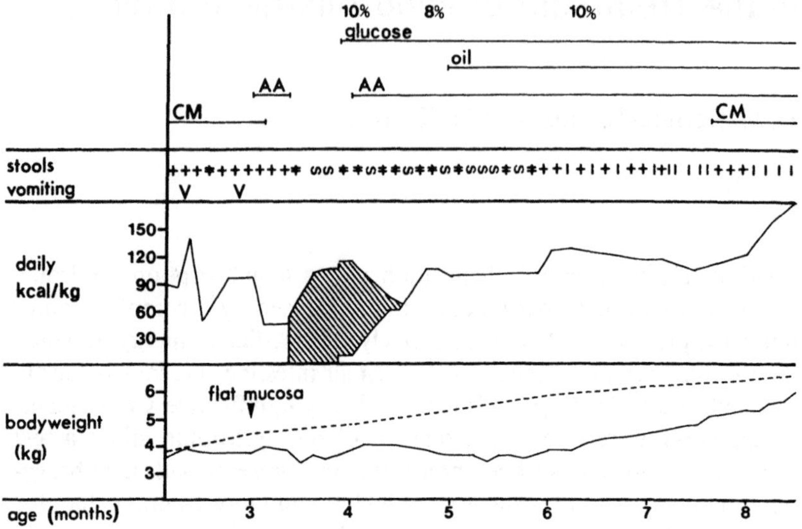

Fig. 1. Clinical course in an infant fed an hyperosmotic formula. Nourishment given was: cow's milk formula (*CM*), amino acids (*AA*), glucose, and oil. *Shaded area*, parenteral nutrition; *dashed line*, third percentile in weight; | normal stools, ∽ watery diarrhea

total α-glycosidase activity of the damaged small-intestinal mucosa can be overtaxed by too large amounts, e.g. 10 g per 100 ml, perhaps causing an osmotic diarrhoea afresh through the bacterial degradation products of malabsorbed starch. The common dietetic formulas in the 1970s were highly osmotic casein hydrolysates, as e.g. Vivonex, Pregestemil and Nutramigen, the ingredients of which were inadequate according to our experience and opinion today.

Figure 2 draws attention to the point that the calculated amount of calories are not necessarily absorbed through the gut. A very emaciated infant received first of all a parenteral nutrition of 120 kcal/kg body weight and clearly developed satisfactorily, although this amount of calories was not particularly high. This situation appeared to be stable under pure human milk feeding. Maltodextrin was added in order to achieve a better weight gain. Although, in simple arithmetic, the amount of calories was thereby increased, it produced a reoccurence of diarrhoea, most probably because the absorption capacity for this polysaccharide was exceeded. The net absorption of calories by the body must thus have been fewer than calculated. When a casein hydrolysate (Nutramigen) and later, when aged 5 months, a soya milk formula were attempted, neither was tolerated. Both challenges, as well as the rela-

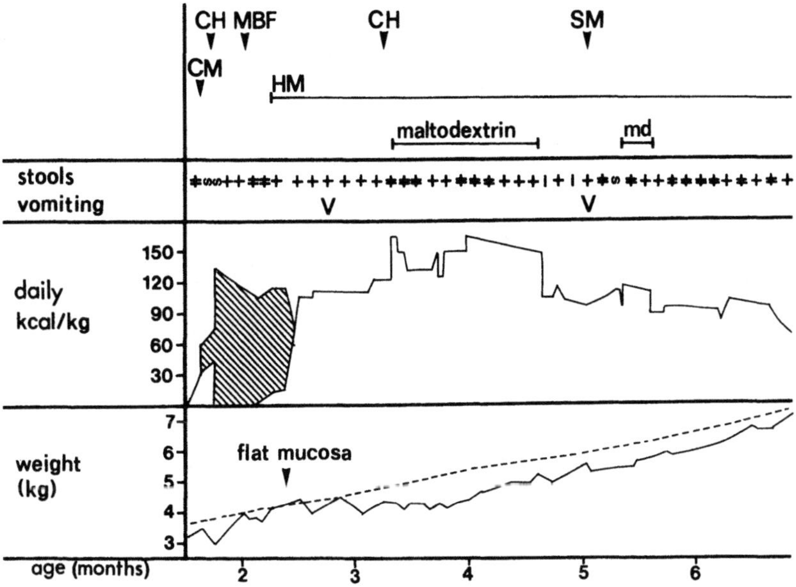

Fig. 2. Clinical course in an infant fed calories that could not be absorbed. Nourishment given was: cow's milk formula (*CM*), casein hydrolysate (*CH*), meat-based formula (*MBF*), human milk (*HM*), maltodextrin (*md*), and soya formula (*SM*). *Shaded area*, parenteral nutrition; *dashed line*, third percentile of weight

tively low supply of calories, certainly contributed to body weight remaining below the third percentile for a long period.

Figure 3 shows one of the most problematic children who ever confronted us. This Turkish infant weighed 4880 g at birth, was fed with a cow's milk formula from the beginning and showed diarrhoea and failure to thrive almost immediately. We had problems with parenteral nutrition, for the child developed one catheter sepsis after the other and was not sufficiently nourished over the parenteral route. Orally administered foods invariably produced strong vomiting. This involved Nutramigen, human milk, and a cow's milk protein hydrolysate. Weight reduced drastically and rapidly without parenteral nutrition. The biopsy of the small intestine showed an unchanged flat mucosa after 5 months of fruitless therapeutic efforts. Therefore, we started prednisone therapy and, in addition, attempted to protect the catheter using a broad antibiotic and antimycotic treatment following a *Candida* sepsis. Every reduction of prednisone, provoked renewed vomiting. Although the small-intestinal mucosa had improved morphologically by the fifth

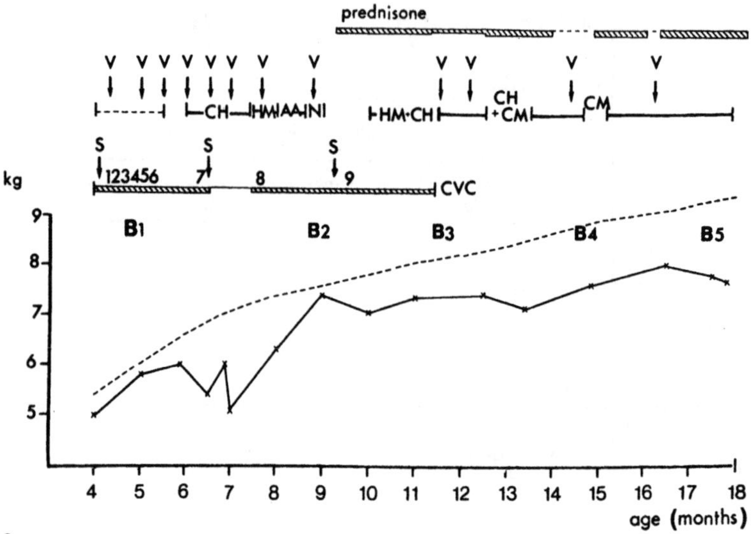

a

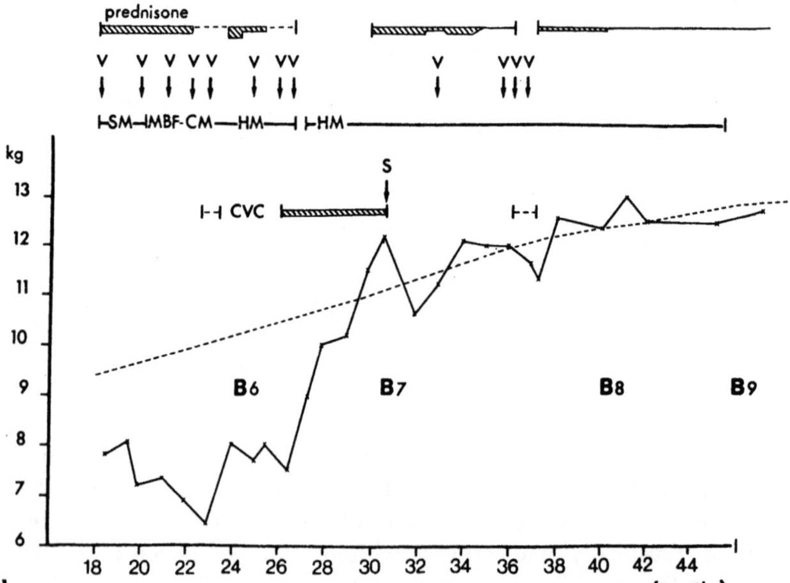

b

Fig. 3a, b. Clinical course in an infant with very strong, multiple reactions over a very long period. **a** Early. **b** Later. Nourishment given was: casein hydrolysate (*CH*), human milk (*HM*), amino acids (*AA*), Nutramigen (*N*), cow's milk formula (*CM*), soya formula (*SM*), and meat-based formula (*MBF*). *CVC*, Central venous catheter; *B*, biopsy; *S*, sepsis; *V*, vomiting. *Dashed line*, third percentile of weight biopsy, growth remained markedly disturbed. The attempt to eliminate steroids and to use other foods, among them a soya formula and a meat-based formula, was met by strong reactions and marked weight loss. The child received central venous feeding again for 2 months when aged 2 years, and, for the first time, weight increased to above the third percentile. Subsequently, body weight developed solely with human milk feeding, initially still with prednisone, roughly along the third percentile. Human milk, without the concomitant administration of steroids, was tolerated only when aged 4 years. In later years, an increasingly purely IgE-mediated food allergy developed to cow's milk protein, with high specific IgE milk antibodies.

The case of this unusual patient makes clear how important the transition from a catabolic to an anabolic situation is for the recovery of the mucosa and for the subsequent tolerance of food, in this case human milk. The steroids certainly could prevent the acute strong reaction and stimulate the recovery of the intestinal mucosa. However, a transition to the anabolic situation was not attained.

The poor experience in the 1970s with highly osmotic hydrolysates, which in addition still released further allergic reactions, made it essential to find new formulas.

At the beginning of the 1980s Nestlé introduced a new hydrolysate (Alfaré) which was interesting particularly in the small size of the protein molecule and its low osmolarity. Since then, further new hydrolysates have become available on the West German market, from which certain important features are summarized in Table 1. The protein source in Alfaré is cow's milk whey; in Pregomin it is a mixture of soya

Table 1. Hypoallergenic formulas (15%)

	Alfaré	Pregomin	Humana HS	Beba HA (13.2%) (Aletemil HA)
Protein source	Cow's milk whey	Soya, beef collagen	Soya, beef collagen, cow's milk whey	Cow's milk whey
Protein content (g/dl)	2.5	2.0	2.1	1.6
Seize of peptides (daltons)	<5000	<5000	<17000	<20000
Carbohydrates (g/dl)				
Maltodextrin	6.7	6.8	7.9	2.2
Starch	0.9	1.8	-	lactose 5.2
Fat (g/dl)	3.6	3.6	3.9	3.4
MCT	1.7	-	1.2	-
Osmolarity (mosmol/l)	200	210	200	240

protein and beef collagen; in Humana HS soya, whey and meat connective tissue; and in Beba HA and Aletemil HA, whey protein. The protein content lies between 2.5 and 1.8 g/dl for the 15% solution. The molecule size is smallest in Alfaré and Pregomin. In the latter, 95% of the peptides have a molecular weight under 2000 dalton. Both Humana HS and Beba HA have large molecular peptides. Beba HA contains only lactose. Alfaré and Humana HS have a large proportion of medium-chain triglycerides. The osmolarity of the milks is equally low, that of Aletemil HA being the highest.

Our experiences with the new so-called hypoallergenic foods are presented in Figs. 4–6. The course of a severely undernourished female infant is shown in Fig. 4, whose body weight increased to above the third percentile following treatment with Alfaré and parenteral nutrition using a central venous catheter. The number of stools declined, and small intestinal morphology and function improved through an increase in disaccharidase activities. The continuation of the Alfaré feeding alone produced no immediate convincing progress, perhaps due to a problem of calories combined with a temporary intestinal infection. An improvement occurred with human milk, which was maintained with the

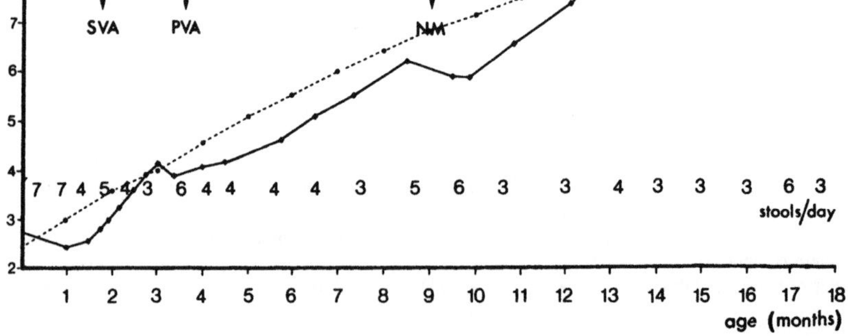

Fig. 4. Clinical course in an undernourished female infant with a flat small-intestinal mucosa fed hypoallergenic formulas. Nourishment given was: Alfaré (*A*), human milk (*HM*), Pregomin (*P*). *CVC*, Central venous catheter; *B*, biopsy; *SVA*, subtotal villous atrophy; *PVA*, partial villous atrophy; *NM*, normal mucosa. *Dashed line*, third percentile of weight

change to Pregomin. An intervening rotavirus infection led to a renewed weight loss. A weight gain was achieved when human milk was reintroduced. The addition of Alfaré and the tolerance of an increased amount finally led to a weight increase above the third percentile. The transition to soya milk, which was readily tolerated, was achieved at age 1.5 years. The intestinal mucosa was normal, both morphologically and in its dissarcharidase activities, i.e. in the Pregomin and human milk phase, already at the age of 9 months.

The next child had trisomy 21 (Figure 5). It should be noted here that four children with Down's syndrome were among our patients with cow's milk allergy and mucosal injury, so that we can confirm the Finnish observation that this form of allergy occurs particularly frequently in such infants.

This child received a complete parenteral nutrition at first for over 2 months with additional human milk. MBF treatment alone was not tolerated, but 15% Alfaré was successful.

Most recently we have turned to making use of hypoallergenic formulas following unsuccessful initial treatment with a lactose- and fat-reduced formula (so-called *Heilnahrung*) over 2–3 weeks in very young infants who were not breast fed and did not recover from acute enteritis, and in whom the development of cow's milk allergy and mucosa injury was suspected.

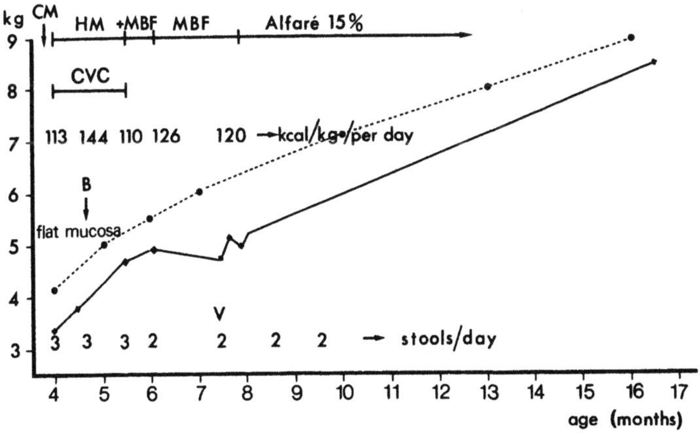

Fig. 5. Clinical course in a male infant with Down's syndrome. Nourishment given was: cow's milk formula (*CM*), human milk (*HM*), meat-based formula (*MBF*), and Alfaré. *CVC*, Central venous catheter; *B*, biopsy, *V*, vomiting. *Dashed line*, third percentile

The following example (Fig. 6) shows such a child who came to us at age 7 weeks and became increasingly dystrophic during the feeding of *Heilnahrung* and evacuated six or seven watery stools per day. Consequently, we began treatment with Pregomin in the 3rd week of treatment and gave a very substantial number of calories, which apparently was not sufficiently absorbed in the 1st week as six watery stools per day were still observed. Starting from the 4th week, a continuous weight increase and recovery was observed up to the 10th week, with distinctly fewer stools. One should pay attention to the essential, enormous amount of calories needed for this weight gain. This calorie requirement is often underestimated. To underline the point once more, although large numbers of watery stools were evacuated with 166 cal/kg at the beginning, indicating that the absorption capacity was exceeded, it is important that it was not accompanied by weight loss or further dehydration due to the low osmolarity of the diet. This means that a worse bowel movement with such a hypoallergenic and, above all, hypoosmotic diet should not be considered disturbing so long as no further weight loss is produced. The transition to a lactose-containing cow's milk formula was readily tolerated starting from the 9th week.

Purely IgE-mediated food allergies are usually easier to treat when only one or two antigens are concerned. Generally it is sufficient to

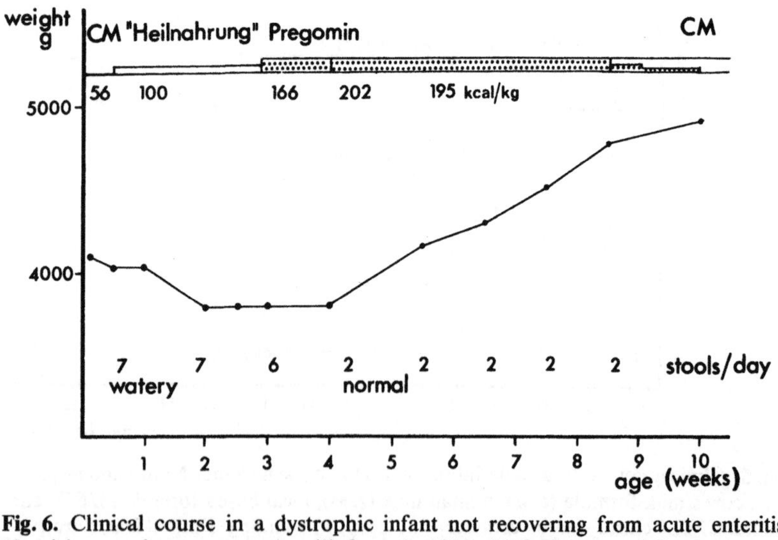

Fig. 6. Clinical course in a dystrophic infant not recovering from acute enteritis. Nourishment given was: cow's milk formula (*CM*), *Heilnahrung* and Pregomin

eliminate selectively the antigens in question from the diet either of the mother, who is breast feeding, or the infant itself. Soya preparations have, without question, their place in this context.

The following example (Fig. 7) shows a child who was exclusively breast fed and developed in this period a generalized and most severe weeping eczema, heavy colic, and slimy diarrhoea, and who had maximally raised IgE values with four-fold positive radioallergosorbent tests (RAST) for egg, milk and fish. Whenever the mother ate fish, this infant reacted immediately with severe diarrhoea. Confronted by this multiple allergy, there was no other choice than to take the infant, aged 6 months, off breast feeding and to substitute a hypoallergenic diet which was by no means well accepted, as was evident in the low-caloric intake. While the eczema improved, growth remained unsatisfactory and the protein, apparently lost through the skin, was insufficiently replaced. Height fell to below the third percentile, although the weight finally showed an improvement with the addition of potatoes and chicken to the diet.

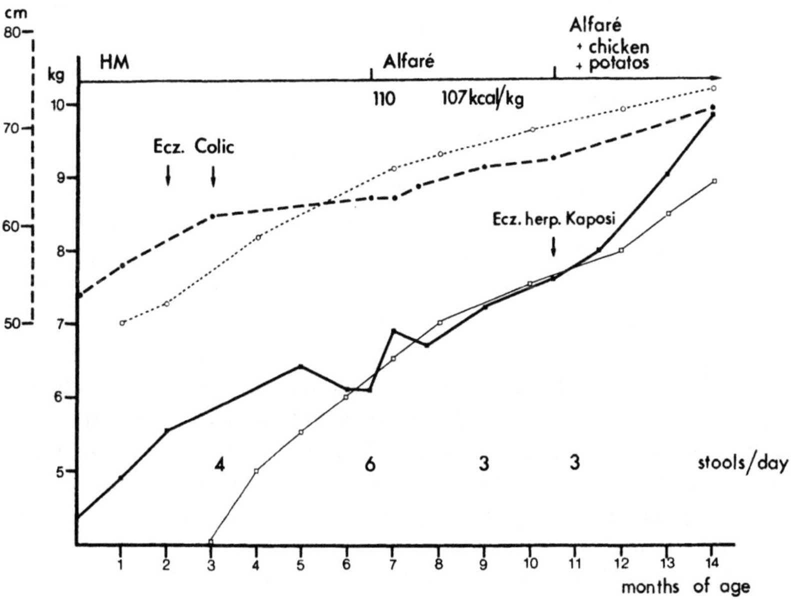

Fig. 7. Clinical course in an infant with multiple allergies fed a hypoallergenic diet. Nourishment given was: human milk (*HM*), Alfaré, chicken, and potatoes. *Dotted line* and *thin solid line*, third percentile

This case, which is certainly a rare exception, was remarkable for us because, firstly, breast feeding was accompanied by a marked weight loss, and, secondly, an unsatisfactory diet was further maintained with the insufficient supply of calories, which apparently was due to the unpalatable taste of the hydrolysate. It is, for us, the single form of an obviously IgE-mediated food allergy which proceeded with such a severe dystrophia. Unfortunately, we were not permitted to conduct a small-intestinal biopsy in this child.

The last example is that of a 5-month-old, exclusively breast-fed infant from an atopic family who developed, starting in the 4th week of life, a pronounced eczema and, in the 6th week, colic. A homeopathic therapist attempted to treat the eczema orally with 4 × 20 ml whey. He thereby released an anaphylactic reaction with marked laryngeal and pharyngeal oedema. Subsequently, the mother attempted to alleviate the symptoms by eliminating cow's milk from her own diet but achieved no improvement. This was not suprising as the infant demonstrated, through its increased IgE, a four-fold positive RAST test, not only to milk protein but also to egg white. Treatment with Alfaré brought an improvement. A first attempt to treat with Beba HA produced the same symptoms as those of the whey challenge from the homeopathic therapist, namely, an acute anaphylactic reaction with heavy swelling of the throat and shortage of breath. We concluded from this that this type of so-called hypoallergenic food is certainly capable of releasing a reaction in those suffering from a cow's milk protein allergy.

In summary, it can be stated that human milk is the most successful diet in cases of severe cow's milk allergy with malabsorption. Unfortunately, the retrovirus catastrophy permits only the application of pasteurized human milk. The new low-osmotic, so-called hypoallergic formulas with low molecular peptides (<5000 dalton) have proved their worth in the treatment of severe cow's milk allergy with mucosal injury. A diet phase over several weeks with a hypoallergenic formula, with low molecular peptides, is to be recommended for every infant under 3 months of age who has not been breast fed, and in whom an acute enteritis persists longer than 2 weeks. Soya milks are not suitable in the treatment of cow's milk allergies with small-intestinal mucosal injury. An attempt is, however, justified to treat a purely IgE-mediated allergy with soya formulas.

If the allergy is released by foreign antigens in the breast milk, an attempt should be made to restrict the antigens in the mother's diet. In cases of multiple allergy, then, under certain conditions, breast feeding must be stopped.

So-called hypoallergenic formulas with higher molecular weight of the protein, e.g. Beba HA, can still release IgE-mediated allergic reactions and cannot, therefore, be unreservedly recommended at the moment.

References

1. Meeuwisse GW (1983) High sugar worse than high sodium in oral rehydration solutions. Acta Paediatr Scand 72:161–166
2. Sandhu BK, Jones BJM, Brook CGD, Silk DBA (1982) Oral rehydration in acute infantile diarrhoea with a glucose-polymer electrolyte solution. Arch Dis Childh 57:152–154

Sodium Cromoglycate in the Management of Food Allergy in Children

L. Businco, A. Cantani, P. Meglio, and P. G. Giampietro

Introduction

Children with disorders related to adverse reactions to foods are frequently a puzzle for allergists as regards both diagnosis and therapy. It is assumed that food allergens stimulate mediator release from the superficial mast cells located in the gut, thereby inducing an increased permeability of the gastrointestinal (GI) tract. Food protein absorption into the blood stream ensues, which is followed by atopic manifestations at distant sites, such as angioedema, atopic dermatitis (AD), urticaria, asthma, and GI symptoms, the latter being provoked by the effects on the gut itself. It has been shown by experimental models that local anaphylaxis is associated with increased GI porosity to the antigens present in the gut lumen and is at the same time the triggering agent [1].

The treatment of choice in such disorders is avoidance of the offending foods. This can be easily achieved when the child is allergic to foods which are not common items in the diet, such as strawberries, sea foods, citrus fruit, peach, etc., or when the offending food is not a necessary nutrient, such as apples, nuts, chocolate, etc. Problems arise, however, when the child is allergic to foods which are common items in the diet or which have important nutritional value (cow's milk, eggs, fish, etc.). In these cases a drug capable of preventing symptoms would be useful in order to avoid a strict diet free of such important nutrients. Sodium cromoglycate (SCG), the salt of a bischromone carboxylic acid, is of proven efficacy in the prophylaxis of bronchial asthma and other disorders associated with mast cell degranulation. The drug has different modes of action, such as inhibition of rat passive cutaneous anaphylaxis and the antigen-induced histamine release from passively sensitized peritoneal cells [2]. More recently, clinical studies have indicated that SCG has a direct effect on inflammatory cells, inhibiting various leukocyte functions (membrane receptor expression, cytotoxic capacity) and in vitro activation of human neutrophils, eosinophils, and monocytes [3, 3a].

The aim of the present study is to review the literature on the use of SCG for the management of food allergy (FA) in children.

Clinical Studies

Laboratory Data

SCG is able to significantly reduce the absorption of macromolecules, apparently inhibiting mediator release from the sensitized mast cells in the gut mucosa. In six patients slightly sensitive to egg, a reduction both in the amount of serum ovalbumin and in symptoms was observed after SCG administration [4, 5]. Several studies have reported on the use of SCG in FA patients in whom food produces immune complexes. In all these studies, oral SCG prior to food challenge prevented both the symptoms and formation of the complexes [6–9].

To evaluate the intestinal permeability in 22 children, half of whom were allergic and half healthy, the 6-h urinary recovery of differently sized polyethylene glycols was measured before and after SCG administration. While no difference was noted between the two groups before the trial, after SCG was given a significant decrease in uptake was observed in the FA children. Permeability properties of the affected children thus seemed to return to normal after SCG treatment [10].

Sugar absorption has recently been employed as a diagnostic tool in various GI disorders. Normally, lactulose is not absorbed by the GI mucosa, whereas mannitol crosses it. Measurements of urine mannitol and lactulose have therefore been performed as noninvasive means of evaluating the state of the GI mucosa in celiac disease and of diagnosing FA [11]. In FA patients a reduction in mannitol absorption and an increase in lactulose absorption have been demonstrated after challenge tests [12]. It has recently been shown that 300 mg SCG in water solution 15 min before challenge with the offending food is able significantly to reduce the absorption of lactulose and to increase the absorption of mannitol [2].

These clinical data, taken together, strongly suggest that SCG acts by inhibiting mast cell gut degranulation, thus preventing tissue injury.

Table 1. Studies on the management of food allergy in children

Authors	Year	*n*	Age	Design	Dose (mg/day)	dos/k	Duration (months)	Disease	ST	RAST	Challenge	Evaluation	Efficacy
Freier, Berger [14]	1973	4	5	O	200		<1	Urt	+	ND	O	Cha	+
Blanckaert et al. [15]	1975	1	1	O	NR			Urt	ND	ND	O	Cha	+
Shaw [16]	1975	1	6	O	NR			AD	ND	ND	O	Cha	+
Esteban et al. [17]	1977	4	0.5	O	600		>12	Mult	+	+	O	Cha	+
Freier [18]	1977	30	0.8	S	150		<1	Urt	ND	ND	O	Cha	–
Molkhou, Waguet [19]	1979	39	0.5–12	O	100–600		<1	AD	ND	+		Cha	+
Businco et al. [20]	1980	20	2–4	O	NR	30	<1	Asth	+	+	O	Cha	+
Cavagni et al. [21]	1981	13	1–9	O	800		1–3	AD	+	+	O	cl	+
Atherton et al. [22]	1982	30	2–10	D	400		1–3	AD	ND	ND		Cha	–
Molkhou, Waguet [23]	1982	40	NR	D	200–800		1–3	AD	ND	ND		Cha	+
Businco et al. [24]	1983	10	3–14	S	NR	30	<1	Mult	+	+	S	Cha	+
Harris et al. [25]	1983	29	7	O	100–200		1–3	AD	+	+	D	cl	?
Giannetti et al. [26]	1984	11	1–14	D	NR	40		AD	ND	ND		cl	+
Graham et al. [27]	1984	29	3–12	D	NR		3–6	AD	–	+		cl	+
Boner et al. [28]	1985	28	0.5–9	O	200–1600		1–3	AD	ND	ND		cl	+
Corrias et al. [29]	1985	20	0.5–10	S	NR	40	1–3	AD	+	+		cl	+
Erwin, Jones [30]	1985	1	7		100		3–6	Mult	+	+		Cha	+
Businco et al. [31]	1986	31	0.5–10	D	400–1600		1–3	AD	+	+	O	Cha	+

O, open; S, single-blind; D, double-blind; Urt, urticaria; AD, atopic dermatitis; Mult, multiple; Asth, asthma; ST, skin test; RAST, radioallergosorbent test; Cha, challenge; cl, clinical diagnosis; dos/k, dosage per kg; NR, not reported; ND, not done

Clinical Data

Although SCG has been widely used for the management of respiratory allergy, conflicting results of FA treatments have been reported by several authors [13]. In FA patients it has been shown, for instance, that SCG acts in the GI tract rather than after absorption into the blood stream. SCG pretreatment of a soy-allergic patient gave no protection when the drug was inhaled, whereas oral treatment with 400 mg blocked either the immediate or the late reaction [14].

There have been 17 papers published in English on the management of FA in children [14–31] (Table 1). The studies covered 331 children aged 0.5–12 years. Of these, 11 studies reported on 271 children aged 0.5–12 years who were affected with AD (Table 2); four were carried out open, i.e., without blinding, one employed a single-blind design, and four a double-blind design. The dosage of SCG used was not reported in five studies; in the 12 remaining trials daily doses (in milligrams) were: 100, 150, 200, 100–200, 100–600, 400, 600, 800, 200–800, 200–1600, and 400–1600. The duration of the trial was less than 1 month in four studies, between 1 and 3 months in seven, between 3 and 6 months in two, and longer than 1 year in one; in three it was not reported. Four of the five open studies yielded positive results, i.e., confirming SCG as an effective means for the management of AD; the double-blind studies were positive in three cases and negative in two. The only study with doubtful results was one conducted in an open design. Table 3 shows the relationship between study design and SCG effectiveness in 60 children aged 0.5–7 years affected with other allergic diseases. No study was carried out in a double-blind fashion. Four open studies showed positive results, the other one negative results.

Table 2. Study design and SCG effectiveness in 271 children (0.5–12 years) with atopic dermatitis

Results	Study design			
	Open	Single-blind	Double-blind	Total
Negative	–	–	2	2
Doubtful	1	–	–	1
Positive	4	1	3	8
Total	5	1	5	11

Figures represent number of studies.

Table 3. Study design and SCG effectiveness in 60 children (0.5–7 years) with food allergy (urticaria, asthma, diarrhea)

Results	Study design			
	Open	Single-blind	Double-blind	Total
Negative	–	1	–	1
Doubtful	–	–	–	–
Positive	4	1	–	5
Total	4	2	0	6

Figures represent number of studies.

In summary, 8 of 9 open studies, 2 of 3 single-blind studies, and 3 of 5 double-blind studies gave positive results, while 1 of 2 single-blind and 2 of 5 double-blind studies yielded negative results. Results were doubtful only in one open study.

Tables 4 and 5 and Fig. 1–6 illustrate the results of two studies of our own in 41 children with FA aged 3–12 [23, 31]. The prerequisite for enrolling children in these trials was that they showed positive response to elimination-provocation tests and positive skin tests and radioallergosorbent tests (RAST) to the offending food(s). Tables 4 and 5 summarize the clinical data and symptoms of eight children allergic to cow's milk (CM) and five to egg, before and after administration of 30 mg/kg SCG per day for 7 days. Pretreatment with oral SCG prevented allergic reactions effectively in 6 of 8 CM-sensitive children (Table 4). SCG also prevented the development of untoward reactions to foods in 4 of 5 egg-sensitive children (Table 5) [23].

Figures 1–3 show the results of a double-blind crossover trial with oral SCG in 31 children with AD due to FA [31]. The children under study were divided into two groups: those receiving first SCG and then placebo (group 1) and those receiving first placebo and then SCG (group 2). Analysis of the two groups showed marked differences. Figure 1 shows the variations in clinical assessment of eczema (on a scale from 0 to 240) by the clinician at each clinic visit using body diagrams. Among patients in group 1 (Fig. 1a) there was no statistically significant difference between treatments, although there was a trend in favor of SCG at the end of the challenge period. Among patients in group 2 (Fig. 1b), however, there was a significant difference between treatments in favor of oral SCG at the end of the diet period ($p<0.05$). Figure 2 shows the total daily diary card scores (scale, 0 to 12) for each

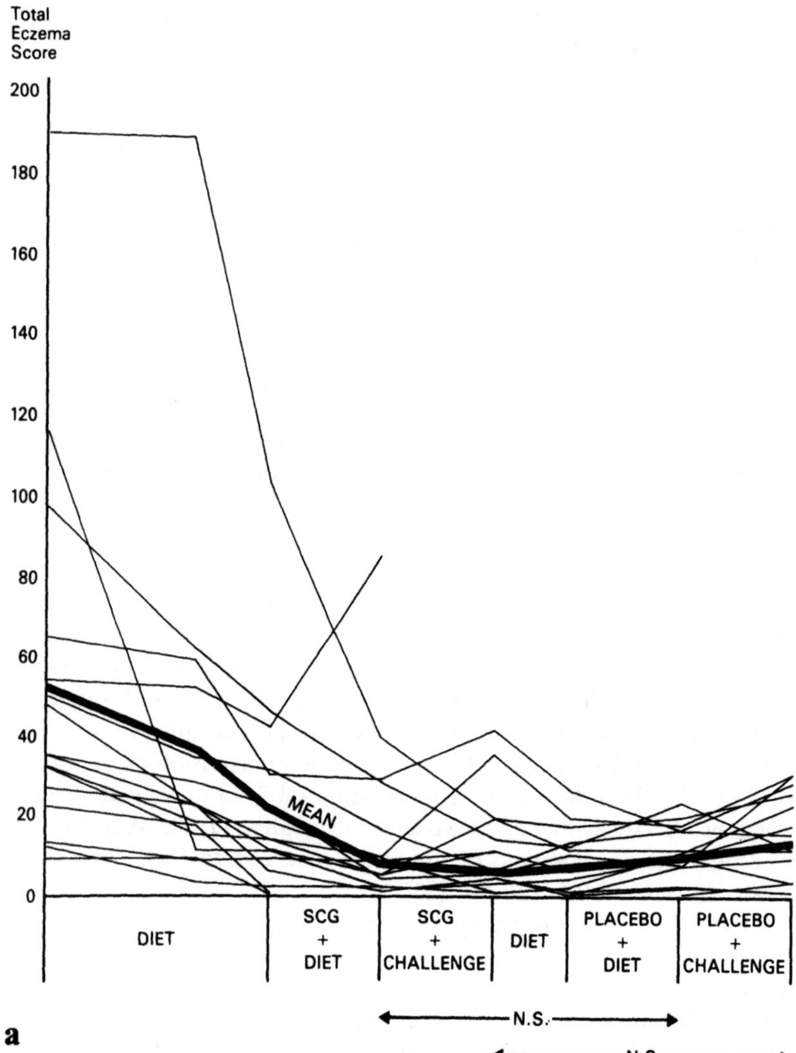

Fig. 1a. Total eczema scores, as assessed by clinicians. **a** Patients receiving first SCG, then placebo (group 1)

treatment phase as assessed by parents. In group 1 (Fig. 2a) there was no significant difference between treatments. In group 2 (Fig. 2b), on the other hand, at the end of the elimination diet period there was a

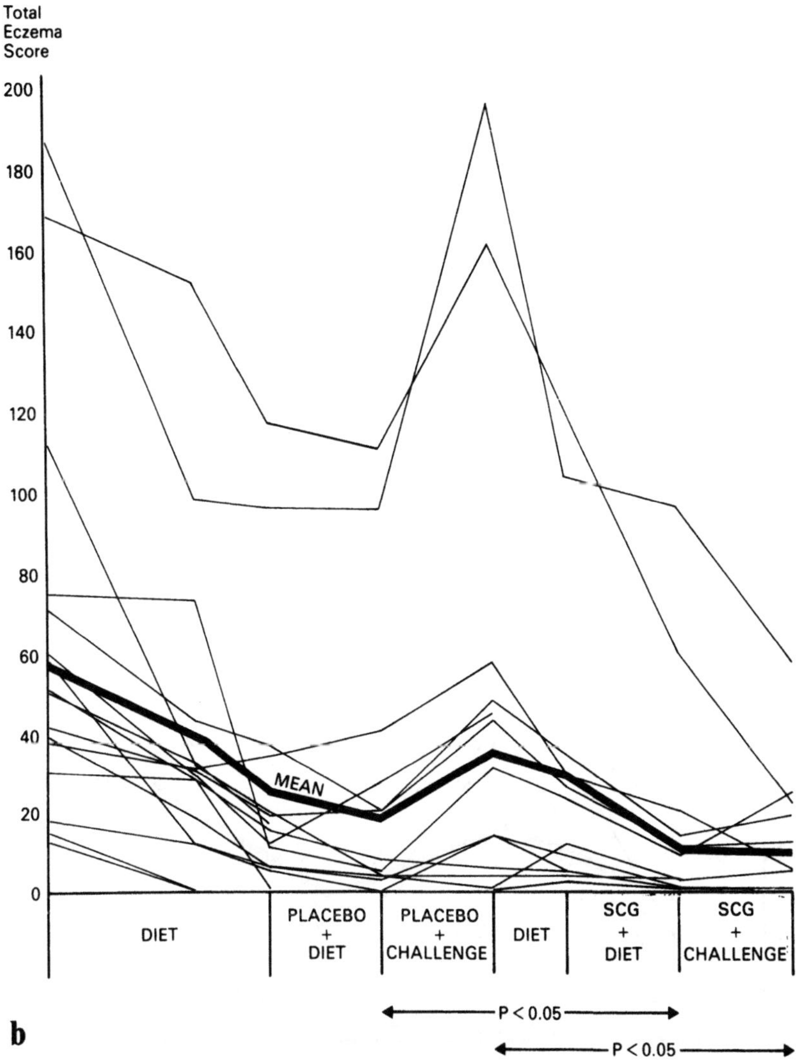

b

Fig. 1b. Patients receiving first placebo, then SCG (group 2)

significant difference in favor of SCG ($p < 0.01$), as there was the end of the challenge period ($p < 0.01$).

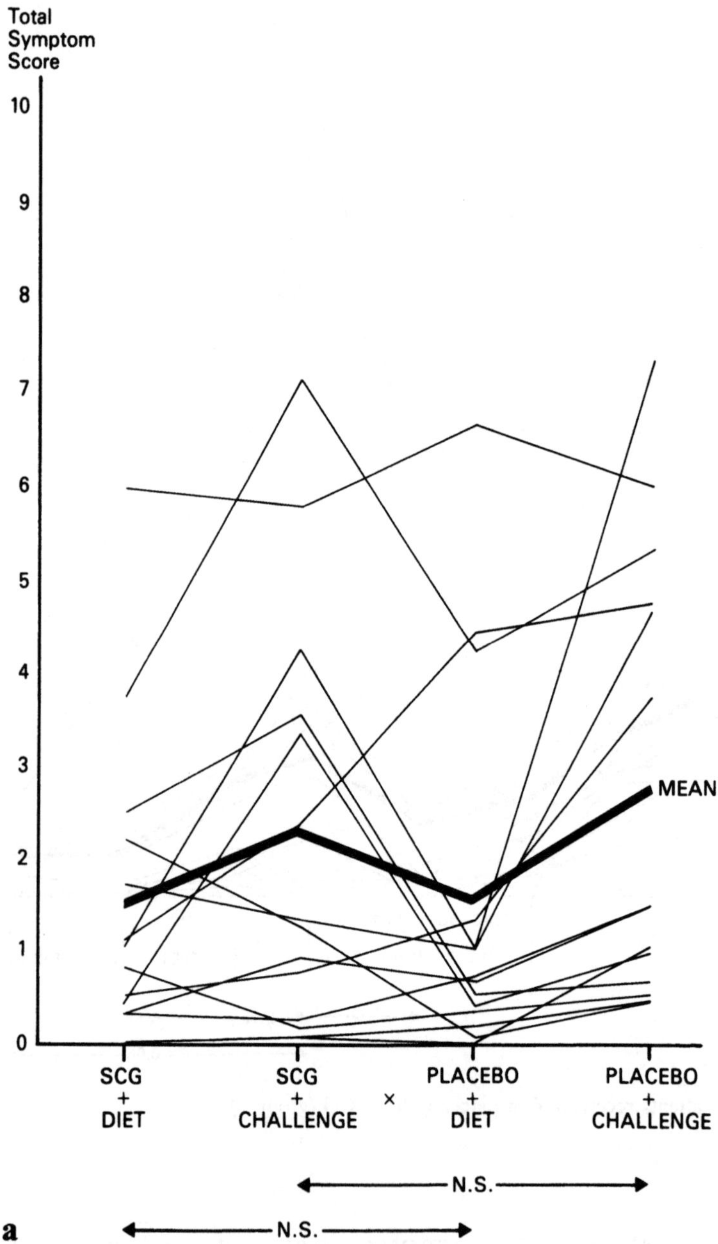

a

Fig. 2a. Total symptom scores, as assessed by parents. **a** Patients receiving first SCG, then placebo (group 1)

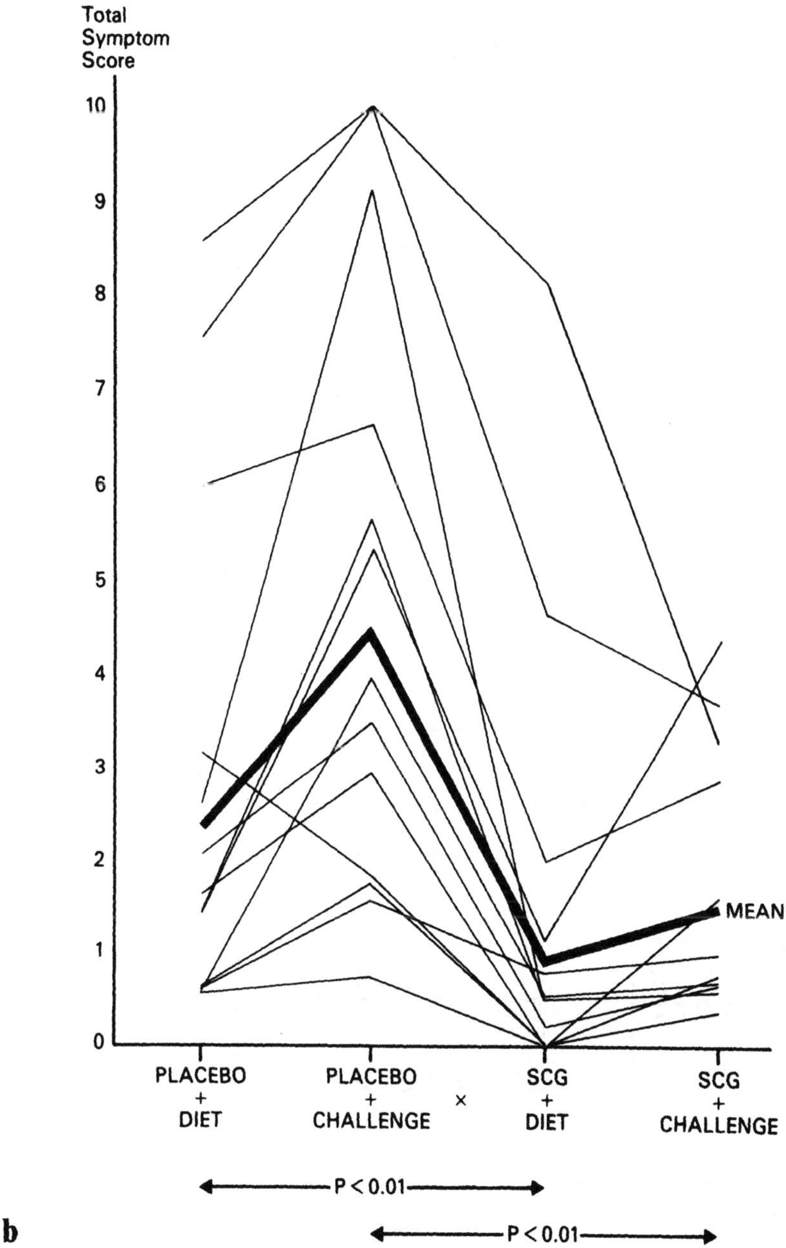

Fig. 2b. Patients receiving first placebo, then SCG (group 2)

Table 4. Clinical data and symptoms before and after 30 mg/kg daily SCG administration for 7 days (milk-sensitive children)

Patient	Age (years)	Sex	Specific IgE to cow's milk (PRU/ml)	Skin test	Prausnitz-Küstner test	Skin window	Symptoms before SCG	Time to onset (min)	Symptoms after SCG
GC	5	M	17.5	+++	+++	+	Asthma	8	–
UR	8	M	17.5	+++	+++	+	Urticaria Lip's edema	2	–
MM	7	M	17.5	+++	+++	+	Asthma Diarrhea Urticaria	2	Asthma
CM	11	M	17.5	+++	++	+	Asthma	8	Asthma
CL	12	M	5.4	+++	+++	+	Asthma	10	–
FS	6	F	5.4	+++	+	+	Asthma Lip's edema	12	–
DF	14	M	1.8	++	++	+	Diarrhea Edema of tongue	8	–
CC	6	M	5	+++	+	+	Urticaria Diarrhea Lip's edema	8	–

Table 5. Clinical data and symptoms before and after 30 mg/kg daily SCG administration for 7 days (egg-sensitive children)

Patient	Age (years)	Sex	Specific IgE to cow's milk (PRU/ml)	Skin test	Prausnitz-Küstner test	Skin window	Symptoms before SCG	Time to onset (min)	Symptoms after SCG
DM	3	F	17.5	+++	+++	+	Urticaria Asthma	15	Urticaria
DA	7	M	5.4	+++	+	+	Diarrhea Eczema Asthma	7	–
UR	8	M	10	+++	+++	+	Asthma	15	–
CL	12	M	17.5	+	+	+	Asthma	5	–
FS	6	F	9.5	+++	++	+	Asthma	13	–

Considering all patients together and both means of assessment – clinician assessment by body diagrams and parent assessment by diary cards – there was an overall significant difference between oral SCG and placebo during both the diet phase and the challenge phase of the trial. The best overall clinical assessment of eczema status was at the end of the treatment period of oral SCG with an elimination diet (mean, 9.5), which was significantly better ($p<0.05$) than that at the end of placebo and elimination diet period (mean, 13.3). At the end of the challenge phase, oral SCG had proven to be significantly better (mean, 7.7) than placebo (mean, 22.5) in preventing the symptom exacerbation caused by the food reintroduction ($p<0.01$; Fig. 3 a). The same situation applies to the analysis of parents' daily diary cards. Overall, the combination of oral SCG and elimination diet (mean, 1.19) showed itself significantly better ($p<0.05$) than that of placebo and elimination diet (mean, 1.9) in lowering symptom scores (Fig. 3 b). There were no

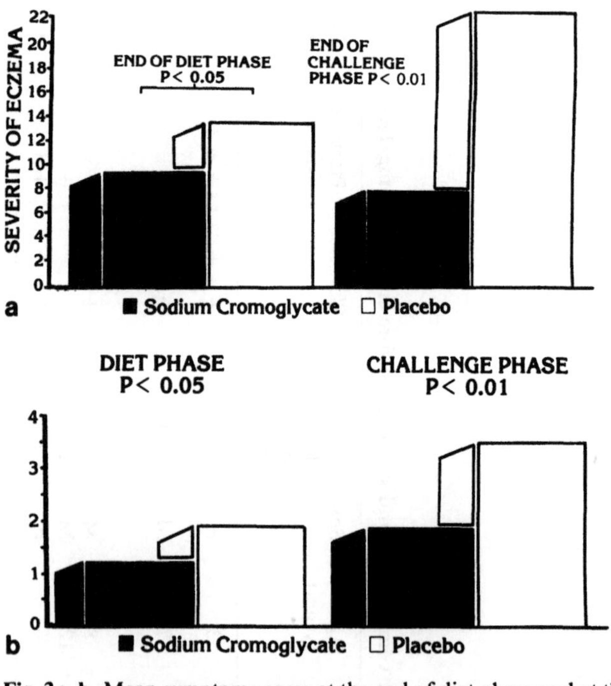

Fig. 3 a, b. Mean symptom scores at the end of diet phase and at the end of challenge phase while children were receiving either SCG or placebo. **a** Severity of eczema scores, as assessed by clinicians. **b** Symptom scores, as assessed by parents

significant differences between the two treatments regarding the other parameters tested (use of test medications, antihistamine usage, and other symptoms).

At the end of the trial and before the design was disclosed, both parents and clinicians recorded their opinions as to which treatment they considered to be more effective (Table 6). There was a significant difference in favor of SCG in the sequence of placebo followed by SCG (group 2). Concerning clinicians' opinions, there was a significant difference in favor of SCG for both groups as well as overall; the difference was highly significant ($p < 0.001$) for group 2 and overall.

Discussion

There have been a number of publications on the use of oral SCG in children with AD and/or FA, several of which have yielded doubtful or negative results [18, 22, 25]. The data in the present study, however show the drug to be effective in the prevention of IgE-mediated FA.

As already reported by previous studies, there are several explanations for conflicting results on SCG in FA. The discrepancy in observations may be due to a number of factors, such as different selection criteria of patients, wide variations in daily dosage of SCG used by various investigators, different amounts of food antigens ingested by the patients during the trials as a result of varying diets followed, diversity in the evaluation of SCG efficacy, problems regarding patient compliance, and the estimation of side effects.

Another possible cause of conflicting results regards differing study designs. Many studies, for example, have employed widely varying SCG dosages. A dose in the range of 30–50 mg/kg per day seems to be most effective. Several studies yielding doubtful or negative results employed much lower SCG doses [18, 22, 25], and this may have prevented

Table 6. Final assessment: patient's/parent's and clinician's opinion

	Parent's opinion	Clinician's opinion
Oral sodium cromoglycate more effective	16	21
Placebo more effective	4	2
Both effective	5	0
Neither effective	1	3
Significance (binomial test)	$p < 0.01$	$p < 0.001$

a (more) positive result. Regarding treatment schedules, SCG was administered in some trials when patients were following an elimination diet, in others when they were on a normal unrestricted diet. Since SCG exerts its action only by way of prevention, its use in patients given widely differing diets may meet with varying degrees of success. This may explain why ATHERTON et al. [22] failed to obtain positive results, since one cannot evaluate the amount of food antigens ingested by children on a normal diet.

Differing evaluation of SCG efficacy may also yield controversial results. An evaluation based upon challenge tests is more objective than a clinical evaluation that encompasses many variables, such as the severity of lesions, the varying extention of body area involved, and the subjective view of the investigator.

Conflicting results can also arise when compliance of either the parents or the children is required. When SCG is available in the form of capsules, children may object that they find them difficult to swallow. An alternative calls for capsules to be dissolved in hot water and diluted in a half cup of cold water or suitable liquid, with the instruction that the resulting drink be swilled around the mouth so that the buccal mucous membrane is coated before the drug is swallowed; however, if this procedure is to be repeated four times a day before meals, a whining child or a frustrated mother may give way to frequent omissions. The child may find it difficult to follow such complicated modalities, and the mother may neglect the schedule due to the strain of housework. Moreover, most children attend nursery schools between the ages of 2 and 4, and these institutions cannot ensure special therapies. Tea parties and picnics are also typical occasions for omissions. The most disquieting issue in this regard is that almost no such omissions are reported to the inquiring doctor.

Standardization of SCG administration would undoubtedly favor complete compliance either of patients or of parents. Finally, SCG generally appears to be a safe drug, and reports of adverse reactions to it are scarce. It should be stressed, however, that children who are to be treated with SCG should be strictly selected according to well-defined criteria. Children should be preselected to assess whether they have definitive clinical and immunological features to assess whether they have definitive clinical and immunological features of IgE-mediated FA, and whether they are affected by food intolerance. It is not recommended to embark up on SCG treatment for a wide spectrum of vague symptoms loosely ascribed to FA; one must also avoid raising false hopes and unrealistic patient expectations.

References

1. Kilshaw PJ, Stade HL (1980) Passage of ingested protein into the blood during gastrointestinal hypersensitivity reactions: experiments in the preruminant calf. Clin Exp Immunol 41:475
2. André C, André F, Colin L et al. (1987) Measurement of intestinal permeability to mannitol and lactulose as a means of diagnosing food allergy and evaluating therapeutic effectiveness of disodium cromoglycate. Ann Allergy 59:127
3. Kay AB, Walsh GM, Moqbel R et al. (1987) Disodium cromoglycate inhibits activation of human inflammatory cells in vitro. J Allergy Clin Immunol 80:1

3a. Skendinger M, Augustine NH, Morris EZ et al. (1987) Effect of disodium cromoglycate on neutrophil movement and intracellular calcium mobilization. J Allergy Clin Immunol 80:573

4. Dannaeus A, Inganas M, Johansson SGO et al. (1979) Intestinal uptake of ovalbumin in malabsorption and food allergy in relation to serum IgG antibody and orally administered sodium cromoglycate. Clin Allergy 9:263
5. Dannaeus A, Johannsson SGO (1979) Prevention of antigen absorption in food allergic patients with oral sodium cromoglycate. In: Pepys J, Edwards AM (eds) The mast cell: its role in health and disease. Pitman Medical, Bath, p 447
6. Brostoff J, Carini C, Wraith DG et al. (1979) Production of IgE complexes by allergen challenge in atopic patients and the effect of sodium cromoglycate. Lancet 1:1268
7. Paganelli R, Levinsky RJ, Brostoff J, et al. (1979) Immune complexes containing food proteins in normal and atopic subjects after oral challenge and effect of sodium cromoglycate on antigen absorption. Lancet 1:1270
8. Brostoff J, Carini C, Wraith DG (1983) The presence of immune complexes containing IgE following food challenge and the effect of sodium cromoglycate. In: Proceeding on the second Fisons food allergy workshop, Harrogate, January 19–21. The Medicine Publishing Foundation, Oxford, p 30
9. Brostoff J, Carini C (1983) Regulation of IgE complex formation in food allergic subject. Proc XII Cong Eur Acad Allergol Clin Immunol, Rome, September 1983. O.I.C. Medical Press, Firenze p 33
10. Falth-Magnusson K, Kjellmann N-IM, Magnusson K-E et al. (1984) Intestinal permeability in healthy and allergic children before and after sodium cromoglycate treatment assessed with different-sized polyethyleneglycols (PEG 400 and PEG 1000). Clin Allergy 14:277
11. Pearson ADJ, Eastham EJ, Laker MF et al. (1982) Intestinal permeability in children with Crohn's disease and coeliac disease. Br Med J 20:285
12. André C, Colin L, Descos L et al. (1984) Non-invasive evaluation of intestinal permeability in food allergy, coeliac disease and inflammatory bowel diseases. Gut 25:1189
13. Dahl R (1978) Disodium cromoglycate and food allergy. The effect of oral and inhaled disodium cromoglycate in a food allergic patient. Allergy 33:192
14. Freier S, Berger H (1973) Disodium cromoglycate in gastrointestinal protein intolerance., Lancet i:913
15. Blanckaert D, Pont JL, Farriaux JP (1975) Utilisation per voie orale du cromoglycate disodique dans le traitement de l'allergie alimentaire. Lille Méd 20:646
16. Shaw RF (1975) Cromolyn therapy in chronic infantile eczema. Arch Dermatol 3:1537

17. Esteban MM, Ojeda Casas JA, Laso Borego MT et al. (1977) Oral disodium cromoglycate in food allergy. Acta Allergol 32:413
18. Freier S (1977) A therapeutic trial of disodium cromoglycate in gastrointestinal allergy. Acta Allergol 13 (Suppl): 109
19. Molkhou P, Waguet JC (1979) Oral disodium cromoglycate in the treatment of atopic eczema in children. In: Pepys J, Edwards AM (eds) The mast cell: its role in health and disease. Pitman Medical, Bath, p 617
20. Businco L, Perlini R, Pacifico L et al. (1980) The value of sodium cromoglycate (SCG) in the prevention of food allergy. Ann Allergy 44:57
21. Cavagni G, Paganelli R, Rigoli E (1985) SCG effect on macromolecular absorption of food antigens in atopic dermatitis (AD). Pediatr Res 19:1119
22. Atherton DJ, Soothill JF, Elvidge J (1982) A controlled trial of oral sodium cromoglycate in atopic eczema. Br J Dermatol 106, 681
23. Molkhou P, Waguet JC (1982) Atopic dermatitis in children and food allergy. Mechanisms of action or oral sodium cromoglycate. 2nd International symposium on immunological and clinical problems of food allergy, Milan, Italy, Oct 1982
24. Businco L, Cantani A, Benincori N (1983) Efectiveness of oral sodium cromoglycate (SCG) in preventing food allergy in children. Ann Allergy 51:47
25. Harris JM, Graham P, Hall-Smith SP et al. (1983) The use of sodium cromoglycate and exclusion diets in childhood atopic eczema. Proceedings of the second Fisons food allergy workshop. Harrogate, Jan 19–21. Medicine Publishing Foundation, Oxford, p 111
26. Giannetti A, Lembo G, Zanoletti T et al. (1984) Il disodiocromoglicato (DSCG) nella dermatite atopica. G Ital Dermatol Venereol 119:365
27. Graham P, Hall-Smith SP, Harris JM et al. (1984) A study of hypoallergenic diets and oral sodium cromoglycate in the management of atopic eczema. Br J Dermatol 110:457
28. Boner AL, Valletta EA, Antolini I et al. (1985) Trattamento della dermatite atopica con sodiocromoglicato in bambini non selezionati per allergia alimentare. Minerva Pediatr 37:262
29. Corrias A, Rossi G, Orani S et al. (1985) Terapia con DSCG nell'allergia alimentare dell'infanzia. Minerva Pediatr 37:453
30. Erwin A, Jones JR (1985) Oral cromolyn sodium in milk induced anaphylaxis. Ann Allergy 54:199
31. Businco L, Benincori N, Nini G et al. (1986) Double-blind crossover trial with oral sodium cromoglycate in children with atopic dermatitis due to food allergy. Ann Allergy 57:433

Food Allergy – Epidemiology and Prediction

N.-I. M. Kjellman

Food allergies are common during childhood (Table 1) [1, 2] and are closely related to current or later developing atopic disease (bronchial athma, allergic rhinitis, allergic urticaria, atopic eczema and certain gastrointestinal syndromes). The accumulated prevalence of atopic diseases is approximately 26%–30%, as reported in recent studies [3, 4]; their prevalence is probably increasing. Although the symptoms are usually mild or moderate, they may present a threat to the child's psychosocial adaptation. Furthermore, treatment costs for all allergies and atopic diseases are tremendous [5].

These factors have contributed to the interest in identifying risk factors for the development of allergy and atopic disease and of possibilities for predicting their development in order to establish recommendations on their prevention or, at least, the delay of their onset [6]. Risk factors that have been identified are the following (see also in [7]):

- Family history of atopic disease
  - Maternal smoking during pregnancy
  - Maternal intake of β-blocking agents during pregnancy
  - Birth during or immediately prior to inhalant allergen season (pollen or mite)

Table 1. Children with food reactions to any food (total) and to egg and fish during the first 4.5 years of life in 144 children grouped by family history of atopic disease

Family history	Total children	Children with reactions		
		Total	Egg	Fish
Bilateral	48	58	15	13
Unilateral	58	29	14	5
None	38	13	5	0

- Perinatal stress and/or operations
- Early occasional feedings with cow's milk
- Early weaning or supplemental feeding with cow's milk formula
- Maternal allergen intake during the early nursing period
- Smoking in the family
- Early exposure to pets
- Excessive exposure to mites
- Early infections
- Early intake of allergenic foods
- Humid indoor climate
- Heavy air pollution

- Contributing factor
  - Immune deficiency (T cells, IgE regulation)

The modern way of life has been blamed for the increasing incidence of atopic disease, especially through the use of chemicals, possibly acting as adjuvants. Decreased breast feeding and other changes in feeding habits may in part also explain the increase. The introduction of blankets, favouring the growth of mites, is thought to explain the recent increase in bronchial asthma in Papua New Guinea. Indoor and outdoor pollution with irritants may act together with allergens, especially in a person with a high genetic propensity for developing atopic disease or allergy. Infections may disturb the normal immune-regulatory balance, thereby promoting the so-called allergy breakthrough.

Before pregnancy a carefully obtained history offers a fair chance for prediction of atopic disease. The sensitivity of an immediate family history is 49%, and the specificity only 50%, for atopic disease at some point before 7 years of age. This was evaluated in a nonselected population of 1700 children followed up prospectively from birth [3]. A remote family history (found in 58% of the newborn infants) showed considerably lower efficiency as predictor of atopic disease.

IgE determination in expectant parents, especially the mother, may give some information regarding the child's level of IgE at 4 months of age [7], but this is by far inferior to cord blood IgE determination for the prediction of atopic disease. Determination of maternal IgG antibodies to food allergens has also been advocated as an allergy predictor [8]. Low concentrations were found especially in mothers of infants with early-developing allergic symptoms when fed the corresponding allergen. However, our own studies, with blind evaluation of children at 18 months of age, could not confirm a long-term predictive value of maternal IgG antibody determination [9].

High concentrations of IgE in cord blood are highly predictive of subsequent food sensitization, especially against hen's egg. The value of cord blood IgE determination as a predictor of atopic disease has been confirmed in almost all studies. Cord blood IgE has a moderate sensitivity (40%) regarding atopic disease at some age during the first 7 years of life, but it has a high specificity (94%) and thus a higher efficiency than family history (71% versus 63%). The most important finding is that long-term atopic disease, i.e. reported to be present at all four follow-up occasions, seems to be identified already at birth in 94% of the 91 cases with such long-term disease.

Several other tests are currently being evaluated for their predictive capacity.

Hence, there is enough evidence of extrinsic factors involved in the development of atopic disease to give us reason to search for ideal tests or combinations of tests to find candidates at high risk for allergy or atopic disease. The best available test is IgE determination combined with a carefully obtained family history.

References

1. Kjellman N-I M (1983) Development and prediction of atopic allergy in childhood. In: Boström H, Ljungstedt N (eds) Theoretical and clinical aspects of allergic diseases. Skandia International Symposia. Almqvist and Wicksell, Stockholm, pp 57–73
2. Andersson JA, Sogn DD (1984) Adverse reactions of foods. AAAI and NIAID report, NIH Publication no 84-2442
3. Kjellman N-I M, Croner S (1984) Cord blood IgE determination for allergy prediction - a follow-up to seven years of age in 1651 children. Ann Allergy 53:171
4. Hattevig G, Kjellman B, Björkstén B, Johansson SGO (1987) The prevalence of allergy and IgE antibodies to inhalant allergens in Swedish school children. Acta Paediatr Scand 76:349-355
5. Hjalte K, Croner S, Kjellman N-I M (1987) Cost-effectiveness of neonatal IgE-screening for atopic allergy before 7 years of age. Allergy 42:97–103
6. Wahn U, Seger R, Wahn V (1987) Pädiatrische Allergologie und Immunologie. Fischer, Stuttgart
7. Hamburger RN (1984) Diagnosis of food allergies and intolerance in the study of prophylaxis and control groups in infants. Ann Allergy 53:673–677
8. Casimir G, Gossart B, Vis HL (1985) Antibody against beta-lacetoglobulin (IgG) and cow's milk allergy. J Allergy Clin Immunol 75:206
9. Fälth-Magnusson K, Kjellman N-I M, Magnuson K-E (1988) Antibodies IgG, IgA and IgM to food antigens during the first 18 months of life in relation to feeding and development of atopic disease. J Allergy Clin Immunol 81:743–749

Prolonged Exclusive Breast-Feeding as a Determinant of Infantile Atopy and Infections

E. Savilahti, V.-M. Tainio and L. Salmenperä

Human milk is the best nutrition for the full-term infant during the first months of life. It also has advantages which cannot be compensated by artificial feeding methods, such as the physical closeness of the mother and infant. While the nutritional needs of the infant can be met sufficiently by a well-balanced formula, the non-human proteins in the formula provoke immune reactions in the infant, and formulas lack the protective agents, particularly secretory IgA, of human milk [1]. Several studies [2–8] have suggested that breast-fed infants have less frequent atopic symptoms than those who are weaned early. This has been disputed, however [9, 10], particularly in more recent studies [10–15] and in the present study [16]. In a prospective nutritional study on 198 infants [17] we carefully recorded all signs of atopy and infections and studied the interrelations with feeding regimes.

Patients and Methods

Participants were recruited among mothers who had given birth to healthy babies at the Department of Obstetrics of the University of Helsinki. The goal was to obtain 200 newborn infants for the study. Two families dropped out during the 1st year. The infants visited the paediatric clinic at 2, 4, 6, 9 and 12 months of age. We provided all medical care during the 1st year of life. At the mean age of 2.3 years, parents of all infants were asked to complete a questionnaire about the health of their infant during the 2nd year of life. Fifteen families failed to return the questionnaire.

Feeding. We encouraged mothers to continue exclusive breast feeding as long as possible in order to study its nutritional value. The number of exclusively breast-fed infants gradually fell to 101 by the age of 6 months and to 31 by the age of 9 months [17]. Infants were weaned on an adapted formula with 16 g/l protein. Fruit and vegetables were added at the age of 3 months, cereals and meat at 5 months. Thirty-one infants were completely weaned by 3.5 months; they were all breast fed from birth, exclusively for a median of 11 days and partially for 70 days.

Atopy. We diagnosed atopy if the infant had any of the following features:

- Pruritic dry dermatitis, consisting of erythema or papules outside the nappy area and present on two or more visits during the 1st year of life.
- A history of urticarial eruption.
- Three or more episodes of wheezy bronchitis during the 1st year.
- Three or more of the following symptoms: rhinorrhoea for more than 1 month; itching or watering eyes; gastrointestinal symptoms provoked by foods; one or two wheezy bronchitis attacks during the 1st year.
- Dermatitis described by the parents to be compatible with atopic eczema during the 2nd year of life.

Statistical Analysis. The χ^2 and *t* tests were used for comparisons. The predicting factors for atopy were analysed by stepwise logistic regression. The following predictor variables were tested: 1. education of mothers; 2. size of home; 3. type of day-care (period of more than 6 months during the 2nd year); 4. heredity for atopy; 5. age at first exposure to cow's milk (formula); 6. age at start of regular formula feeding; 7. total duration of breast feeding; 8. age at introduction of solid foods; and 9. number of respiratory tract infections during the 1st year. The predictor variables were treated in the first analysis either as continuous (variables 2, 5, 6, 7, 8, 9) or categorical (variables 1, 3, 4); in further analyses all variables were treated as categorical.

Results

Atopic Manifestation. Fourteen infants (7% of total) had signs of atopy during the 1st year, and a further 31 (17%) had signs suggestive of atopy during the 2nd year. Only three infants had symptoms of asthma.

Logistic regression analysis showed heredity for atopy to be the only statistically significant risk factor for predicting the occurrence of atopy

($\chi^2=4.33$, df=1, $p<0.05$; Table 1). Exclusive breast feeding lasting more than 6 months was a probable risk factor for atopy ($\chi^2=3.44$,

Table 1. Risk factors for atopy (logistic regression analysis)

	Relative risk	
	95% Confidence interval	p
Heredity for atopy	1.41 1.00–1.98	<0.05
Exclusive breast feeding >6 months	1.37 0.96–1.96	<0.1

The other seven variables tested were not statistically significant.

Table 2. Atopy in groups with varying duration of exclusive or total breast feeding, in infants with heredity for atopy, and in groups with different frequency of respiratory infections

Group	Number of children	Percent with atopy appearing during 1st year of life ($n=198$)	Percent with atopy appearing during 2nd year of life ($n=183$)
Short-term breast feeding (<3.5 months)	31	0[b]	13
Long-term exclusive breast feeding (>9 months)	31	16[b]	15
>6 months exclusive breast feeding[a]	101	7	23
Heredity for atopy	79	9	24[c]
No heredity for atopy	119	6	10[c]
Frequency of upper respiratory tract infections during the 1st year			
High (⩾6)	53	9	10
Moderate (3–5)	103	6	15
Low (0–2)	42	7	22

[a] Median length of exclusive breast feeding was 278 days; most infants were fully weaned after the age of 12 months.
[b] $p=0.02$.
[c] $p=0.04$.

Table 3. Frequency of atopy during the first 2 years of life according to duration of exclusive and total breast feeding and heredity for atopy in selected groups of infants

Type of feeding	No heredity for atopy			Heredity for atopy		
	No atopy	Atopy		No atopy	Atopy	
	(*n*)	(*n*)	(%)	(*n*)	(*n*)	(%)
Short-term total breast feeding (<3.5 months)	18	1	5%[a]	9	3	25%
<6 months breast feeding	26	4	13%	12	3	20%
>6 months exclusive breast feeding	47	12	20%	30	13	30%
Long-term exclusive breast feeding (>9 months)	13	5	28%[a]	9	4	31%

[a] $p = 0.06$

Table 4. Feeding of infants with or without atopy

Group	Lenght of exclusive breast feeding	Age when regular formula was started	Age when breast feeding was stopped	Age at the introduction of solid foods
1st-year atopy	250	304	309	231
2nd-year atopy	210	214	234	205
Atopy (collapsed)	220	235	250	205
Non-atopics	179	203	246	189

Figures represent number of days.

df = 1, $p < 0.1$). More infants in the long-term exclusively breast-fed group than in the short-term breast-fed group showed atopy during the 1st year of life (Table 2). The number of infants with and without heredity for atopy was similar in both groups (13 in long-term and 12 in short-term breast-fed groups; Table 3).

More infants with heredity for atopy had signs of atopy during the 2nd year than those without heredity ($p = 0.04$; Table 2). The occurrence of atopy did not differ significantly in infants with low, moderate or high incidence of respiratory tract infections (Table 2). Logistic analysis showed that this factor had no significant risk for atopy. None of other seven variables tested, including age at the introduction of solid foods, were risk factors for atopy.

The effect of feeding on the incidence of atopy was seen among infants who did not have a family history of atopy (Table 3). The incidence of atopy was higher in the infants exclusively breast fed for more than 9 months than in the short-term breast fed group ($p = 0.06$; Table 3).

When we compared the mean length of exclusively and total breast feeding in infants with or without atopy, there was no difference (Table 4). The mean age of either group at the introduction of solid foods was also quite similar.

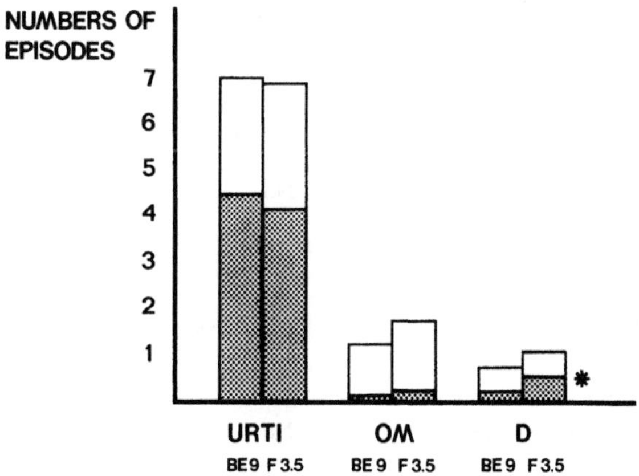

Fig. 1. Mean number of upper respiratory tract infections (*URTI*), episodes of otitis media (*OM*), and diarrhoea (*D*), during the 1st year (*shaded columns*) and the 2nd year (*unshaded columns*) of life. *Left columns*, infants weaned early; *right columns*, infants with prolonged breast feeding. *Asterisk*, $p < 0.05$

Infections. Fewer of the infants with long-term exclusive breast feeding had acute diarrhoea during the 1st year compared to those with short-term breast-feeding (5/31 versus 12/31; $p = 0.06$). The mean number of diarrhoea episodes was also lower (Fig. 1). The number of other infections in these groups was similar (Fig. 1). In the overall study group the mean number of upper respiratory tract infections during the 1st year was 4.3 and during the 2nd year 3.0. The respective figures for otitis media were 0.4 and 1.5 and for diarrhoea 0.4 and 0.6. We analysed the risk factors for recurrent otitis media by logistic regression (Table 5) in the same study group. Long-term breast feeding did not protect against otitis media [18].

The infant's own atopy was a risk factor for recurrent otitis media and was most frequent among those whose otitis presented during the 1st year of life. A high number of child contacts was a particularly important risk factor among those whose recurrence of otitis started during the 2nd year of life.

Discussion

In the present study we found no advantage in prolonging exclusive breast feeding even to 9 months based upon comparison to a group that

Table 5. Potential risk factors for infantile recurrent otitis media (ROM) during the first 2 years of life

	Relative risk (95% confidence interval)	Comments
Frequent upper respiratory tract infections	NS	Most frequent in early onset ROM
Duration of breast feeding	NS	Other three feeding variables also NS
Atopy	1.9 (1.2–3.2)	Most frequent in early-onset ROM
Cow's milk allergy	NS	Otitis media frequent
Type of day-care	NS	Most infants with ROM were outside home
Number of child contacts ⩾5	2.1 (1.3–3.3)	Most contacts in 2nd-year ROM
Smoking of parents	NS	More frequent in infants with ROM

was breast fed for less than 3.5 months. We stress that all infants were initially breast fed in our study, and while we believe that early breast feeding has importance, we were not able to study this.

There are many difficulties in comparing the results of studies concerning infant feeding and atopy. The feeding regimens are not well defined; also the term "breast feeding" may imply either exclusive or partial breast feeding. Artificial feeding regimes differ; in earlier studies home-made cow's milk based formulas or commercial formulas with high protein concentration were used [3–6]. The present formulas with lower protein concentration, as used in this study, may be less antigenic and provoke atopy less frequently then in earlier studies.

Little attention has been paid to the qualitative aspects of breast milk. We found that the total IgA content of colostrum was significantly lower in the milk of mothers whose infants later developed cow's milk allergy compared with samples of mothers with non-atopic infants (Fig. 2) [19]. The levels of cow's milk and β-lactoglobulin-specific IgA antibodies were, however, similar in the two groups. Idiotypic and anti-

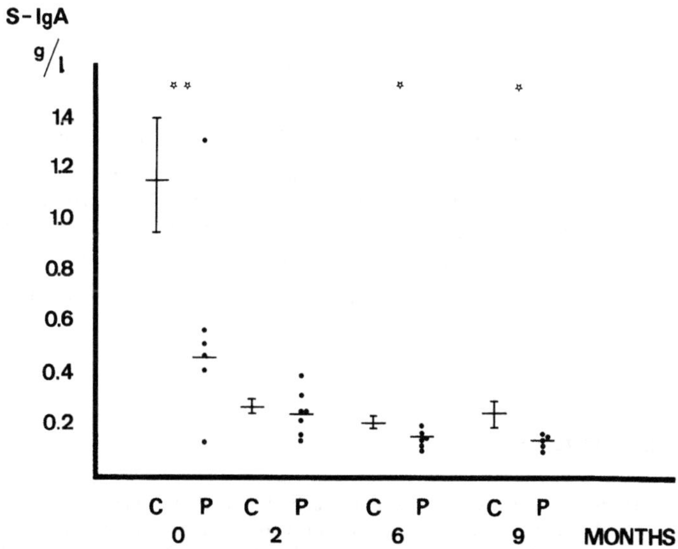

Fig. 2. Concentration of S-IgA in the colostrum and breast milk shortly after delivery, and at 2, 6, and 9 months after delivery. *C*, Comparison groups, 55 non-atopic mothers whose children has no signs suggestive of atopy by the age of 2 years; *P*, mothers of infants who became allergic to cow's milk during the 1st year of life. *Double asterisk*, $p < 0.01$; *single asterisks*, $p < 0.05$

idiotypic antibodies in breast milk may regulate the local immune system of an infant. As the intestine lacks immunoglobulin-producing cells during the first 10 days of life [20], both the protection and modulation offered by breast milk immunoglobulins may be very important, but after the age of 3–6 months, when the local mucosal immune system is better developed [1, 20], breast milk is no longer needed for antigen exclusion.

In our study [16], as in many others [6–13, 15, 21], heredity for atopy was significantly associated with the occurrence of infantile atopy. Earlier studies have suggested that breast feeding is particularly protective against atopy in infants with a positive heredity for atopy [6–8, 15, 21], but we saw no evidence of this. On the contrary, in our study the effect of feeding on the frequency of atopy was seen only among those without such heredity: those with short-term breast feeding had a lower incidence than did those breast fed exclusively over 9 months.

The protection offered by human milk against infectious gastrointestinal infections is well known, particularly in developing countries [2, 10]. We also found that fewer infants on prolonged breast feeding had acute diarrhoea during the 1st year of life than infants put on formula before 3.5 months of age. Whether breast feeding protects against respiratory infections, particularly otitis media, is disputed [2, 10, 22, 23]. We found that none of the feeding variables analysed had an effect on the frequency of these infections [18].

In conclusion, our study showed that in a highly hygienic society prolonged exclusive breast feeding had no advantage over short-term breast feeding with regard to the risk of atopy or respiratory infections during the first 2 years of life. We emphasize that our results may not apply to less developed societies where the incidence of intestinal infections is much higher, and malnutrition of mothers and infants is common.

References

1. Hanson LÅ, Ahlstedt S, Andersson B et al. (1985) Protective factors in milk and the development of immune system. Pediatrics (Suppl) 75:172–176
2. Chandra RK (1977) Prospective studies for the effect of breast feeding on incidence of infection and allergy. Acta Paediatr Scand 68:691–694
3. Grulee CG, Sanford HN (1936) The influence of breast and artificial feeding on infantile eczema. J Pediatr 9:223–225
4. Johnstone DE, Dutton AM (1966) Dietary prophylaxis of allergic disease in children. N Engl J Med 274:715–719

5. Matthew DJ, Taylor B, Norman AP, Turner MW, Soothill JF (1977) Prevention of eczema. Lancet 1:312–324
6. Saarinen UM, Kajosaari M, Backman A, Siimes MA (1979) Prolonged breast feeding as prophylaxis for atopic disease. Lancet 2:163–166
7. Kaufman HS, Frick OL (1981) Prevention of asthma. Clin Allergy 11:549–553
8. Grusky FL (1982) Comparison of breast, cow, and soy feedings in the prevention of onset of allergic disease. Clin Pediatr 21:476–491
9. Halpern SR, Sellars WA, Johnson RB, Anderson DW, Saperstein S, Reisch JS (1973) Development of childhood allergy in infants fed breast, soy or cow milk. J Allergy Clin Immunol 51:139–151
10. Kovar MG, Serdula MK, Marks JS, Fraser DW (1984) Review of the epidemiologic evidence for an association between infant feeding and infant health. Pediatrics 74 (Suppl):615–638
11. Hide DW, Guyer BM (1981) Clinical manifestations of allergy related to breast and cow's milk feeding. Arch Dis Child 56:172–175
12. Kramer MS, Moroz B (1981) Do breast feeding and delayed introduction of solid foods protect against subsequent atopic eczema? J Pediatr 98:546–550
13. Gordon RR, Noble DA, Ward AM, Allen R (1982) Immunoglobulin E and the eczema-asthma syndrome in early childhood. Lancet 1:72–74
14. Fergusson DM, Hoordwood LJ, Shannon FT (1983) Asthma and infant diet. Arch Dis Child 58:48–51
15. Taylor B, Wadsworth J, Golding J, Butler N (1983) Breast feeding, eczema, asthma, and hayfever. J Epidemiol Community Health 37:95–99
16. Savilahti E, Tainio V-M, Salmenperä L, Siimes MA, Perheentupa J (1987) Prolonged exclusive breast feeding and heredity as determinants in infantile atopy. Arch Dis Childh 62:269–273
17. Salmenperä L, Perheentupa J, Siimes MA (1985) Exclusively breast-fed healthy infants grow slower than reference infants. Pediatr Res 19:307–312
18. Taino V-M, Savilahti E, Salmenperä L, Arjomaa P, Siimes MA, Perheentupa J (1988) Risk factors for infantile otitis media: atopy but not type of feeding. Pediatr Res 23:509–512
19. Savilahti E, Salmenperä L, Tainio V-M, Arjomaa O, Simes MA, Perheentupa J (1987) Mothers of infants with cow's milk allergy vs controls have less IgA antibodies to cow's milk protein in milk. Pediatr Res 22:99
20. Perkkiö M, Savilahti E (1980) Time of appearance of immunoglobulin-containing cells in the neonatal intestine. Pediatr Res 14:953–955
21. Kjellman N-I M, Johansson SGO (1979) Soy versus cow's milk in infants with biparental history of atopic disease: development of atopic disease and immunoglobulins from birth to 4 years of age. Clin Allergy 9:347–358
22. Cunningham AS (1977) Morbidity in breast-fed and artificially fed infants. J Pediatr 90:726–729
23. Saarinen UM (1982) Prolonged breast feeding as prophylaxis for recurrent otitis media. Acta Paediatr Scand 71:567–571

Subject Index

GPSR Compliance

The European Union's (EU) General Product Safety Regulation (GPSR) is a set of rules that requires consumer products to be safe and our obligations to ensure this.

If you have any concerns about our products, you can contact us on ProductSafety@springernature.com

In case Publisher is established outside the EU, the EU authorized representative is:

Springer Nature Customer Service Center GmbH
Europaplatz 3
69115 Heidelberg, Germany

Batch number: 10704701

Printed by Printforce, the Netherlands